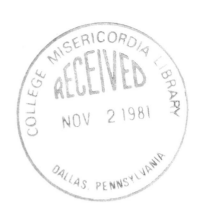

D1716753

Radiological Evaluation of the Spinal Cord

Volume I

Author

Milosh Perovitch, M.D.
The University of Connecticut
School of Medicine
Farmington, Connecticut

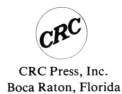

CRC Press, Inc.
Boca Raton, Florida

Library of Congress Cataloging in Publication Data

Perovitch, Milosh.
   Radiological evaluation of the spinal cord.

   Bibliography: p.
   Includes index.
   1. Myelography. I. Title. [DNLM: 1. Myelo-
graphy.] I. Title. [DNLM: 1. Myelography. WL405
P453r]
RC402.2.M94P47   617'.5607'57   80-11454
ISBN 0-8493-5041-7 (v. 1)
ISBN 0-8493-5043-3 (v. 2)

Direct all inquiries to CRC Press, Inc., 2000 N.W. 24th Street, Boca Raton, Florida 33431.

© 1981 by CRC Press, Inc.

International Standard Book Number 0-8493-5041-7

Library of Congress Card Number 78-11454
Printed in the United States

PREFACE

Out of more than 8000 myelographies carried out by the author, about 4000 cases with clinical and/or pathologic information were selected, including 200 spinal cord angiographies, as a basis for the text of *Radiological Evaluation of the Spinal Cord*. The author's intention was to correlate, as much as possible, radiologic findings in spinal cord disorders with their basic clinical and pathologic features. Equally, the purpose of the text was to reflect the essential problems related to the radiologic diagnosis of spinal cord pathology as they are interpreted at present.

The illustrations for the chapter dealing with spinal cord angiography were selected in collaboration with Dr. René Djindjian. The text concerned with gas myelography was considerably enriched through fruitful joint work with Dr. Gerard Gauthier, Professor of Neurology, and Dr. Aloys Werner, Professor of Neurosurgery, Medical Faculty, University of Geneva, Switzerland, who referred their patients to me; and through Dr. Pierre Wettstein, Professor of Radiology, who allowed me full use of the equipment at his Institute of Radiology. Also valuable to this text was my more recent work in the Department of Radiology and the close collaboration with Departments of Neurosurgery and Neurology at the Johns Hopkins University, School of Medicine, and the Johns Hopkins Hospital.

The photographic work for this text was done by Mr. Henri C. Hessels in the Department of Radiology, the John Hopkins Hospital. Mr. Hessels provided the text with illustration of excellent quality on which he worked with great patience and expertise. Most of all, I remain deeply grateful to my wife, Smiljka Perovitch, who did the first redaction of the manuscript.

THE AUTHOR

Dr. Milosh Perovitch received his M.D. degree in 1950 from the University of Beograd, Yugoslavia; Habilitation degree in Neuroradiology in 1958; and his Doctor of Medical Science degree in 1966. He became Board Certified Radiologist in 1954. As a full-time faculty member he headed, from 1954 to 1962, the Service of Neuro- and Vascular Radiology at the Clinic of Neurosurgery, Clinic of Neurology and Cardiovascular Center at the Medical Faculty, University of Beograd. In 1957, Dr. Perovitch carried out advanced studies in neuro- and vascular radiology at the University of Stockholm, Sweden (Karolinska Hospital, Serafimerlazarettet, and Soder Hospital), and briefly at the National Hospital for Nervous Disease, London, England. In 1961, he spent 1 year in the U.S. working on the studies related to advanced radiological diagnostic methods at the Johns Hopkins University School of Medicine, Columbia University School of Medicine, Rochester University School of Medicine, Michigan University School of Medicine, and Stanford University School of Medicine. The studies were sponsored by the U.S. Department of Health, Education and Welfare. In 1962, Dr. Perovitch was appointed Chief, Department of Diagnostic Radiology, at the Radiological Institute, Medical Faculty, Univeristy of Beograd. He continued to head the Service of Neuroradiology and later assumed the responsibilities of the neuroradiologic operation at the University of Geneva, Medical Faculty. In 1968 he became, by invitation, a neuro- and vascular radiologist and full-time faculty member at the Johns Hopkins University School of Medicine, Baltimore.

Since 1971, Dr. Perovitch has been Professor of Radiology, University of Connecticut, School of Medicine. In addition, Dr. Perovitch was Acting Head, Department of Radiology; Head, Section of Neuro- and Vascular Radiology; and Head, Division of Radiological Science at the University of Connecticut, School of Medicine. In 1979, Dr. Perovitch took his sabbatic leave and carried out a research project related to the application of computed tomography and new spinal cord angiographic and myelographic techniques at the Johns Hopkins University; and was a visiting professor at several other universities abroad.

Dr. Perovitch published two books on basic radiology; one chapter dealing with neuroradiological aspects of injuries of the CNS as co-author of the book *Neurotrauma;* and 112 papers, the majority of which are related to neuro- and vascular radiology. He is a member of some national and international societies of radiology, neuroradiology, neurosurgery, neurology, and has been guest lecturer at different universities and meetings.

TABLE OF CONTENTS

Volume I

TABLE OF CONTENTS

Volume II

Chapter 1

EMBRYOLOGY*

A more extensive analysis of the embryology of the spinal cord is not within the scope of this radiologic study. However, an outline of the development of the spinal cord relevant to the further discussion in this text is presented as a complementary introduction.

It seems that the stage of the morula is an adequate form from which the tracing of the formation of the spinal cord could begin. There are two layers of cells that form in the morula and become distinguishable as the trophoblast or the external layer, and the inner cell mass or the internal layer. The proliferation of the inner cell mass leads to the formation of two diverse germ layers, the outer stratum or ectoderm, and the inner stratum or entoderm. The two segments of each germ layer, remaining in mutual contact, form the germ disk, out of which the embryonic disk is developed. The third layer of cells originating from the germ disk and forming into the middle germ layer or mesoderm is situated between the ectoderm and the entoderm in its more advanced phase.[1] The nervous system is born out of the external germ layer or the ectoderm of the embryo.

Despite its complexity, the nervous system has a simple structure in the first stage of its development. The dorsal thickening of the ectoderm forms the neural plate. On the surface of the neural plate, a longitudinal depression appears next, known as the neural groove, that extends along the axis of the embryo. With the further infolding of the ectoderm, the neural groove deepens. In this process, the ectodermal ridges on both sides of the groove become more prominent. They are known as neural folds. The neural folds bend medially until they meet and fuse. Subsequently, the neural groove shapes into the neural tube by the end of the third week of embryonic life. The neural tube is closed all along its length except for its two ends, where the anterior (neuroporus rostralis) and posterior opening (neuroporus caudalis) remain until the end of the 4th week, at which time the embryo reaches the length of 5 mm. The cerebral ventricles and the central canal of the spinal cord derive from the cavity of the neural tube.

Further in its development, the neural tube sinks deeper thus detaching itself from the overlying ectoderm. On both sides of the dorsal midline of the neural tube a proliferation of cells occurs along the residue of the neural folds molding the neural crest (crista ganglionaris) or ganglionic ridge. At first, band-like and attached to the dorsal surface of the neural tube, the neural crest begins separating itself filling the angle between the neural tube and the overlying ectoderm. The band-like appearance of the neural crest becomes segmented due to the formation of the primitive ganglia, and it is here in the primitive ganglia that the sensory fibers of the cerebrospinal nerves arise.[2-4] If the neural tube is not completely fused or detached from the ectoderm, malformations of the nervous system such as spina bifida, myeloschisis, or cranioschisis will occur.[2]

The cephalic part of the neural tube grows wider and it shapes into a large vesicle (archencephalon), the origin of the brain. The primitive vesicle, shortly after its formation, divides into three rudimentary brain vesicles: posterior (rhombencephalon), middle (mesencephalon), and anterior (prosencephalon). On the other hand, the cylin-

* References for this chapter appear at the end of Chapter 2.

dric caudal, the narrower part of the neural tube, generates the spinal cord (medulla spinalis).

If a cross section of the caudal part of the tube is analyzed at this stage, it will show that an abundant proliferation of the cells has occurred and, in consequence, the wall of the primitive cord thickens. This rapid division of cells that actually involves the whole length of the neural tube, changes the inner aspect of the tube by the middle of the 4th embryonic week. There are three recognizable zones around the central canal. The outer marginal layer, almost cell free, forms the white matter of the cord. The middle mantle layer, on the other hand, contains an overflowing quantity of two types of cells: the spongioblasts which develop into neuroglia, and the germinal cells which provide the neuroblasts or predecessors of the nerve cells that form the central gray substance. The internal ependymal layer remains as the ependyma that covers the inner surface of the central canal in the cord and the cavities of the brain.[2-4]

The sulcus limitans, a longitudinal groove, changes the shape of the lumen of the central canal. This rather shallow groove, that can be traced from the cord to the midbrain, is located on each lateral wall of the canal and it represents the margin that divides the substance of the walls into alar and basal laminae. The alar lamina (alar plate) thickens gradually, forming the sensory portion of the gray substance and thus becoming the dorsal gray column. All the motor nuclei emerge from the basal lamina (basal plate) which, as it widens, grows into the ventral gray column. Both alar laminae are fused dorsally by a bridge-like roof plate, whereas the basal laminae are joined ventrally by a floor plate.[2,4]

The internal architecture of the spinal cord consisting of the various components of the nerve tissue gradually becomes distinguishable. The development of the main structural elements that are of interest to us can be concisely described in the following way.

By the end of the 4th week, the intersegmental nerve fibers can be identified in the marginal layer. They arise from the neuroblasts located in the mantle layer. By the 6th week, the primitive dorsal funiculus is apparent in the alar lamina formed by a bundle of fibers originating from the cells in the spinal ganglia. Later, in the 3rd month, the long intersegmental fibers are outlined, and by the 5th month, the corticospinal fibers appear. The central processes of the neuroblasts arising in the spinal ganglia form the dorsal root, whereas the peripheral ones become part of the ventral root.

The process of myelination that influences the functional capacity of the fiber tracts begins in the spinal cord about the 4th fetal month, but it is not completed until the 2nd year of life, or even later (corticospinal tract).[3]

The expansion of different elements of the neural tube is not an even process. Thus, at the beginning, the thickening of the tube varies from one level to the other. The more prominent part forms the segments (neuromeres) of the tube that become evident at the level of the spinal nerves. The segmentation of the tube depends upon the size of the nerves, which is, on the other hand, influenced by the volume of the mesodermal segments or somites to which they are assigned. Later, this segmentation is not apparent on the surface because of the formation of the long projection tracts in the marginal layer. However, the segmental arrangement of the primitive neural tube remains the distinctive characteristic of a formed spinal cord. The structure of different components that originate from the alar and basal laminae can be easily recognized in the cord after birth. The early connections between the spinal nerves and the adjacent mesodermal somites is a permanent association, and the skeletal muscles in their definitive forms are attached to these nerves.[2-5]

Due to the enlargement of the ventral column and funiculus on both sides, the floor plate sinks, and the ventral median fissure appears as a deep groove which remains a final feature of the formed spinal cord.

The spinal cord, which has a cylindric shape, fills the entire length of the spinal canal until the 3rd month of fetal life. It retains almost the same shape through its further development as well as after the complete formation, but a discrepancy regarding the length of the cord and that of the spinal canal begins to show. Namely, the pace of the growth of the canal exceeds the growth pace of the cord. Hence, the cord becomes shorter than the canal, and by the 6th fetal month, it reaches the upper limit of the sacrum. At birth, it extends to the lower border of the third lumbar vertebra. In the adult, it ends about the level of the intervertebral disk between the first and the second lumbar vertebra. The difference in growth between the spinal cord and the spinal canal affects the position and appearance of the spinal nerves within the canal. In the early fetal stage, the nerve roots leaving the cord have a horizontal position and form right angles with the longitudinal axis of the cord. They exit between the edges of the shaping vertebrae. As the growth of the canal becomes faster, the foramina containing the nerves move into a lower position in relation to the levels of the cord. Hence, in order to remain attached to their respective foramina, an elongation of the nerves occurs, especially of those originating from the caudal part of the cord. Further on, this elongation changes the direction of the spinal nerves, and their course, instead of being horizontal, becomes oblique, or almost vertical in the lower part of the canal. In this way, the nerves in the caudal region of the spinal canal form a bundle known as the cauda equina. This explains why the segments, especially those of the lower half of the body, do not share the corresponding level with the spinal cord.[2,4]

Chapter 2

ANATOMY CORRELATED TO THE RADIOLOGIC ANATOMY

I. THE SPINAL CORD AND MENINGES

A. The Spinal Cord and Nerves

The spinal cord forms the elongated part of the central nervous system (CNS) that occupies the vertebral canal. The proximal limit of the spinal cord is determined by the upper border of the anterior arch of the atlas which can be readily established on the radiographs of the cervical spinal canal. However, the anatomic junction between the spinal cord and the medulla oblongata is represented on the surface of the cord by the uppermost rootlet of the first cervical nerve, or by the caudal margin of the pyramidal decussation (decussatio pyramidum), which cannot be recognized accurately on radiologic examinations. The distal limit of the cord reaches the lower edge of the first, or the upper edge of the second, lumbar vertebrae. Yet, the studies done by means of myelographies have demonstrated that these limits can be inconstant. In addition, as mentioned earlier, the spinal cord in children is longer and ends at the level of the third lumbar vertebra.

The weight of the spinal cord is 30 g. Its average length varies from 42 to 45 cm.[4] The length of the spinal cord measured on myelograms (gas myelography) can disclose some variations depending on the position and curves of the spine.

The shape of the spinal cord is rather oval due to the flattening in the ventrodorsal direction, its transverse diameter being longer than the ventrodorsal. This form of the cord can be recognized on the series of gas myelolaminograms (Figure 1).

The spinal cord has two enlargements. The higher one, more prominent, is the cervical enlargement (intumescentia cervicalis). It extends from about the third cervical to the second dorsal vertebrae, and it is created by the greater development of the gray substance that gives rise to the large nerves for the upper limbs. The lower one is the lumbar enlargement (intumescentia lumbalis) from which derive the large nerves of the lower limbs. It stretches from approximately the 9th to the 12th dorsal vertebrae and from there on it becomes narrower and cones into the caudal end of the cord, 1- to 2-cm long, known as the conus medullaris. From the tip of this cone-shaped segment of the cord the filum terminale extends to the coccyx. Its proximal part, the filum terminale interum, about 15-cm long, is surrounded by the nerves of the cauda equina and by the dura mater. Its lower part, the filum terminale externum, projects beyond the nerves and is adherent to the first or second coccygeal vertebra.[4,6]

The cauda equina and the conus medullaris as well as the enlargements of the cord can be outlined on myelograms (Figures 2, 3). Further anatomic properties of the spinal cord are not, however, all recognizable by means of radiologic methods. They will be mentioned here because they can be the site of different pathological processes.

The external surface of the spinal cord is divided by the anterior median fissure (fissura mediana anterior), and by the shallow dorsal median sulcus (sulcus medianus posterior) into the right and left halves. A longitudinal dorsal lateral sulcus (sulcus lateralis posterior) marks the entrance of the posterior nerve roots, and the dorsal-intermediate sulcus (sulcus intermedius posterior) in the cervical and thoracic regions separates the fasciculus gracilis from the fasciculus cuneatus. The last shallow groove on the surface of the cord is the ventral lateral sulcus (sulcus lateralis anterior), the site of attachment of the ventral nerve roots.

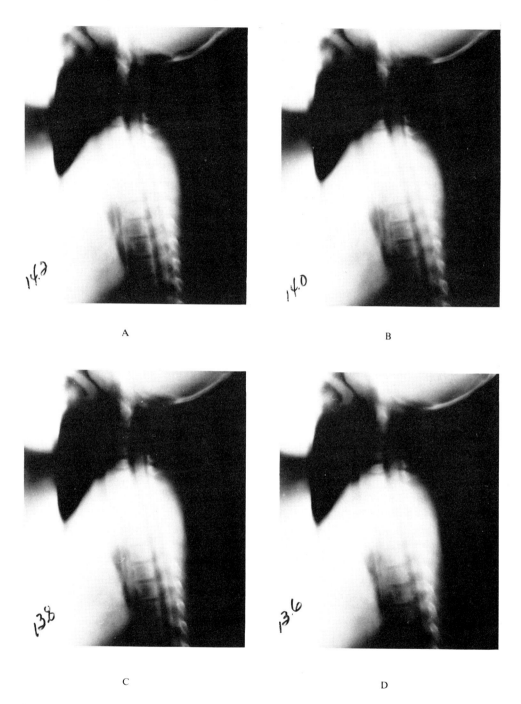

FIGURE 1.   Gas myelograms of an infant showing the changes of the shape of the spinal cord from the midline objective plane 14.2 cm towards the lateral wall of the subarachnoid space (distance between the objective planes is 2 mm on polytomograms).

Along the ventral and dorsal lateral sulcus, the anterior and posterior nerve roots are born out of the spinal cord forming 31 pairs of spinal nerves. Each spinal nerve has an anterior or motor root (radix motoria), and a posterior or sensory root (radix sensitiva). The anterior root is formed by two to three rootlets (fila radicularia) and

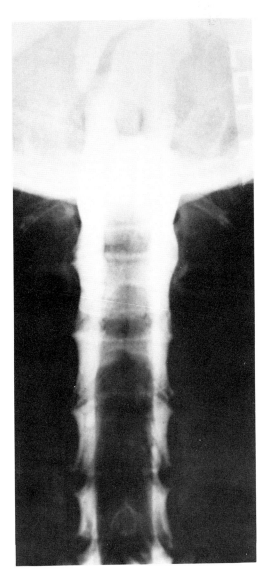

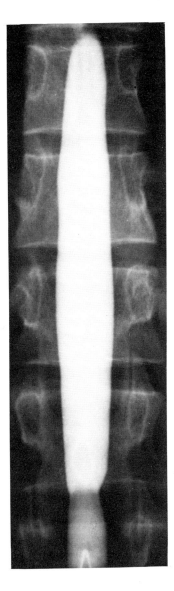

A

B

FIGURE 2(A). Cervical enlargement of the spinal cord. The radiolucency of the dens is seen as well as that of the vertebral artery. The nerve roots surrounded by the meningeal sheaths are outlined. Discreet spondylotic changes at C_5 to C_5 make the roots more apparent. (B) and (C). The flow of Pantopaque® is demonstrated in the upper lumbar and lower thoracic area. The widening of the subarachnoid space is noticeable in the area of lumbar enlargement. The contrast medium appears less radiopaque at the levels of intervertebral spaces in the prone anteroposterior position.

the posterior by six to eight, plus the spinal ganglion (ganglion spinale). According to the segments of the spine, the pairs of spinal nerves are grouped into 8 cervical, 12 thoracic, 5 lumbar, 5 sacral, and 1 coccygeal. The spinal cord itself is divided into three parts: the cervical, thoracic or dorsal, and lumbar. The regions of the spinal cord to which the spinal nerves are attached are referred to as spinal segments (neuromere).[4,6] The beginning of the spinal nerves can be seen clearly on the myelograms with positive contrasts (Figure 4).[7]

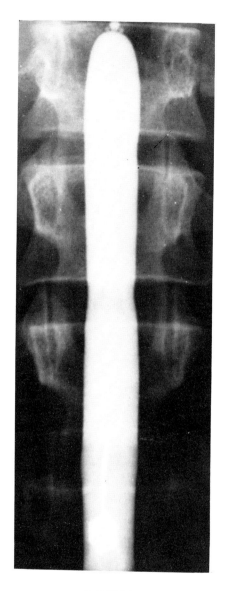

FIGURE 2C.

The central canal stretches along the longitudinal axis of the spinal cord, ending in the filum terminale with an enlargement named the terminal ventricle (ventriculus terminalis). The cephalic end of the central canal is connected to the fourth ventricle. Its diameter is about 0.2 mm, and its cavity is filled with the cerebrospinal fluid (CSF) and lined with ependyma. The central canal represents the primary neural tube.

The inner structure of the spinal cord, as well as the other parts of the CNS, consist of the gray substance (substantia grisea), rich in cells, and of the white substance (substantia alba) where the myelinated and unmyelinated nerve fibers are located. The color of the white substance derives from the myelin.[8]

The white substance surrounds the centrally located gray substance which in the cross section appears as a contour resembling the letter H. The central part of the gray substance that links the two lateral ones is called the central gray substance (substantia grisea centralis), and it consists of gray commissure (commissura grisea) and gelatinous tissue (substantia gelantinosa centralis) placed around the central canal. The lateral

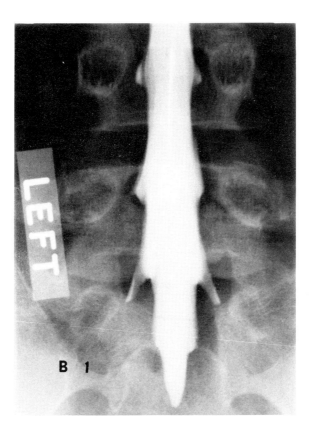

A

FIGURE 3(A). Nerve roots of the cauda equina can be seen on this positive contrast myelogram (Pantopaque®) as fine radiolucent lines. The lower meningeal sleeves are long and wide permitting the nerve roots to be visualized through their exits. The shape and length of the caudal end of the subarachnoid space is well demarcated, and under normal circumstances it can show a number of variations, some of which will be demonstrated on different myelograms further in the text. (B) Oblique view of a myelogram with water-soluble contrast medium (Kontrast U Leo® 20%) outlines the nerves constituting the cauda equina. (C) The gas myelogram shows the lumbar enlargement of the spinal cord, the conus, and the emerging nerve roots (sagittal view).

extension of the gray substance, ventral to the gray commissure, is known as the anterior column (columna ventralis), and the dorsal as the posterior column (columna dorsalis). In the dorsal and upper lumbar regions, a third extension of the gray substance is present. The latter is located laterally to the gray commissure and represents the intermediate lateral gray column. The quantity of the gray matter varies at different levels of the cord.[4,8]

The nerve fibers of the white substance have a longitudinal arrangement. Some of them cross ventrally from one side to the other. The longitudinally displayed fibers form bundles or tracts that perform a certain function. The tracts, functionally closely associated, are the fasciculi.[9] The white matter is divided into the dorsal, lateral, and ventral funiculi.

B. The Meninges

The meninges represent three membranes that extend from the skull into the spinal canal, forming protective sheaths around the spinal cord and the nerves. They are

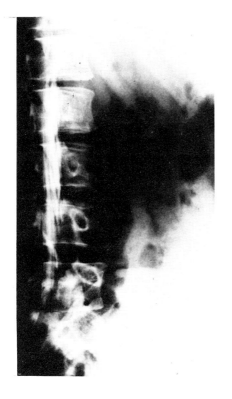

FIGURE 3B.

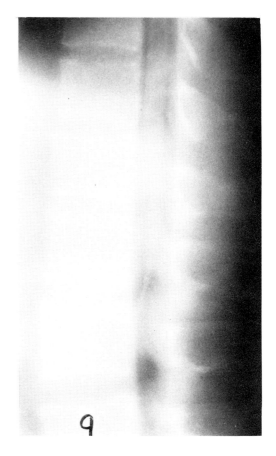

FIGURE 3C.

separated from each other by two concentric spaces filled with fluid. The outer sheath is the *dura mater*, a strong, fibrous membrane adjacent to the bony strucutre of the spine, consisting only of one layer, whereas the intracranial dura mater has two tightly attached layers, the periosteal or outer layer, and the meningeal or inner layer. The outer layer reaches as far as the foramen magnum, but it does not follow the cord in the spinal canal. It actually continues from the foramen magnum as the periosteum of the vertebrae. The inner layer is the one that forms the spinal dura mater. It has the shape of a tube fixed cranially around the foramen magnum, the second and third vertebrae, and to the posterior longitudinal ligament. It is fairly detached and spacious in the lower cervical and lumbar regions, and less loose in the dorsal area. The spinal dura spreads caudally to the second sacral vertebra. At this level it is separated from the anterior wall of the spinal canal and from there on it adheres firmly to the filum terminale, and it ends blending with the periosteum at the dorsal surface of the first coccygeal segment. The dura extends around the spinal nerve roots through the intervertebral foramina. These extensions are shorter and more hoirzontal in the cervical, and longer and oblique in the dorsal and lumbar regions. The first cervical nerve roots coated with the dura can assume an upwards direction.[4,6]

The next meningeal sheath situated between the other two is the *arachnoid*. It is a fine avascular membrane representing the continuation of the intracranial arachnoid into the spinal canal. It surrounds the spinal cord and the cauda equina approximately up to the second sacral vertebra. The arachnoid, like the dura mater, envelops the spinal nerves with their roots forming sleeves around them which can be filled with

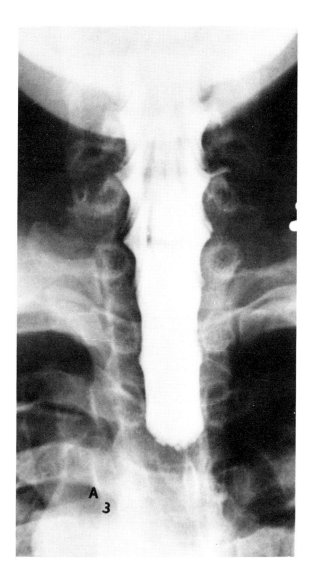

FIGURE 4. Pantopaque® myelogram in the prone anteroposterior position of the patient reveals the cervical spinal cord
with the emerging nerve roots which can be followed to their
exits. The meningeal sleeves are also visible.

positive contrast media. In this way, the spinal nerve roots lodging in these sleeves can
be clearly outlined on myelograms.

The third inner membrane consisting of delicate connective tissue, named *pia mater*,
covers the spinal cord. It is the continuation of the intracranial pia mater, only thicker.
The pia mater is rich in blood vessels that supply the spinal cord, in contrast to the
poorly vascularized dura and avascular arachnoid. The spinal pia mater has two layers.
The internal layer is attached to the spinal cord. Ventrally, it molds into the anterior
median groove, an infolding that brings the blood supply to the nervous tissue of this
region. The external layer of the pia is composed of longitudinally displayed fibers of
connective tissue. These fibers along the anterior median fissure form the linea splen-
dens, and those aligned along each lateral side of the cord make the denticulate liga-

ment. The denticulate ligament is located between the anterior and posterior nerve roots. The part of the subarachnoid cavity of the spinal canal, ventral to this ligament, is known as the anterior compartment and the dorsal as posterior. This ligament has 21 points of attachment with the inner surface of the dura, beginning with the foramen magnum and ending at the conus medullaris. They represent short extensions of the ligament, about 2-cm apart, located between the spinal nerves. Thus the free segments of the lateral border of the denticulate ligament have the shape of an arch whose concavity is turned outside, their whole lateral margin being of a serrate or dentate appearance. The CSF circulates between these insertions from one compartment into the other. In the cervical and thoracic regions, the dorsal subarachnoid compartment is divided into two smaller ones by a posterior septum.[4,10]

Myelography can demonstrate the denticulate ligament. Its radiographic appearance may be helpful in the studies of the movements and the position of the spinal cord, as well as in the delineation of some pathologic processes.

C. The Subarachnoid Space

This space seprates the arachnoid from the pia mater. It communicates directly with the intracranial subarachnoid space. It is a rather wide cavity filled with CSF. In the region of the dorsal junction of the intracranial and spinal subarachnoid spaces, an enlargement is formed, interposed between the lower margin of the cerebellar hemispheres and the medulla oblongata. This is the cisterna cerebellomedullaris or cisterna magna, which is the site of the injection of the contrast medium following the cisternal puncture. The needle is introduced between the occipital bone and the atlas. In the sagittal projection on myelograms, the cisterna magna has an approximately triangular shape (Figure 5).

The caudal part of the subarachnoid space is the location for the lumbar puncture, and the common place for the injection of the contrast media. It varies considerably in size and shape. The tracings from the myelograms collected by Shapiro illustrate various types of the caudal arachnoid sac.[11]

The anterior compartment of the subarachnoid space containing anterior nerve roots is wider in the upper cervical region and triangular in shape. Lower down, it becomes narrower. The posterior compartment containing posterior roots is not clearly outlined on myelograms because the spinal cord is closer to the posterior wall of the spinal canal.

D. The Subdural Space

The subdural space is a narrow fissure separating the dura mater from the arachnoid. This space is filled with a colorless lymph-like fluid. The caudal end of the subdural space differs considerably in size, shape, and length. It can end at the level of the lower border of the fifth lumbar vertebra, or extend to the third or fourth sacral vertebrae. It can be quite wide, or slit-like, diverticular, or rounded.[4,10] Contrast material used for myelographies can be injected into the subdural space if the needle is not inserted far enough into the subarachnoid space, or if this space is shallow or compressed. The subdural injection of a contrast medium often gives an odd picture.

E. The Epidural Space

The epidural space is interposed between the dura mater on one side, and the posterior surface of the vertebral bodies, intervertebral disks, and the posterior longitudinal ligament on the other. It contains connective and fat tissues as well as a plexus of rather large veins. Anteriorly, the extradural space in the cervical region is mostly represented by a fissure. It becomes more spacious in the lower thoracic region, and

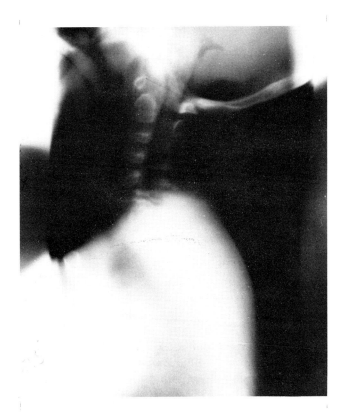

FIGURE 5. Gas myelogram of an infant demonstrates the cisterna magna and pontis, including the fourth ventricle and the cervical spinal cord.

especially in the lumbosacral regions. Posteriorly, it is noticeably wider along the spinal canal, except for the sacral region where the width of the epidural space, both ventrally and dorsally, appears to be the same. The dura mater is attached by connective fibers to the anterior and posterior walls of the canal. The fat tissue accumulated in the lower part of the epidural space can affect the width of the subdural space in obese patients. In this case, the puncture of the subarachnoid space as well as the interpretation of myelograms may prove to be more difficult.[4,7,11]

F. The Ligaments

The bony walls of the spinal canal, intervertebral disks, and the ligaments can affect the radiologic appearance of the spinal cord, nerve roots, or the spaces circumscribed by the meninges.

The bony vertebral canal is wide in the cervical region, the transverse diameter being longer than the sagittal. The canal is of a triangular shape, and the spinal cord normally has enough space on both lateral sides. The canal becomes narrower and rounded in the thoracic region, and again wider and close to a triangular shape in the lumbar area. Such alterations of the contour and size of the bony canal bear an influence on the diameters of the spinal cord, its position, and aspect.[12] The anterior wall of the canal is formed first by the posterior longitudinal ligament, and then ventrally by the posterior surface of the vertebral bodies and intervertebral disks.

The posterior longitudinal ligament is made up of two layers of dense fibers. It runs from the axis to the sacrum, covering the dorsal side of the vertebrae and intervertebral disks. Its cephalic end continues towards the clivus as the membrana tectoria. The ligament is thicker in the thoracic region, and broader in the cervical area.

The transverse ligament of the atlas keeps the dens in contact with the ventral arch. It is a strong ligament which, with its extensions, forms the cruciate ligament of the atlas. These ligamentous structures cover the upper cervical segment of the spinal canal and protrude into its cavity.

Myelograms can demonstrate both ligaments, especially if gas myelography is used. The thickening of these ligaments can be the cause of cord compression and displacement. Furthermore, congenital anomalies of the odontoid such as hypoplasia or aplasia, will cause considerable hypertrophy of the longitudinal ligament with a possible compression of the anterior subarachnoid space and the spinal cord. Often, under these circumstances the cord will be displaced to one or the other side of the canal. Gas myelography can put these changes into evidence. Two more ligaments are important for the radiologic evaluation of this region: the alar or odontoid ligament, and the apical or dental ligament. They limit the rotation of the skull and support the odontoid in its normal position.

The anterior longitudinal ligament covers the ventral surface of the vertebrae and the intervertebral disks from the axis to the sacrum. The anterior and posterior longitudinal ligaments assist the spine in its physiological movements protecting it from dislocations that result from different types of traumas. In this way, indirectly, they shield the structures within the spinal canal.

The intervertebral disks are important components of the anterior wall of the spinal canal. They may be the source of the compression of the spinal cord, its nerves, or meninges. The posterior normal bulging under the ligament, or the pathologic expansion of the intervertebral disks, can be readily detected by myelography. The lateral walls relevant to the contents of the spinal canal consist of pedicles, posterior intervertebral joints, and ligamenta flava. The posterior aspect of the canal is formed by the laminae and the ligamenta flava. From the axis to the sacrum, the laminae of the adjacent vertebrae are connected by the ligamenta flava. They are inserted in the anterior surface of the upper lamina, and in the dorsal surface and the cranial margin of the lower lamina.

The spinous processes of the vertebrae are helpful as points of orientation in regard to the different levels of the spinal canal for a more accurate radiologic determination of the site of the pathologic alterations and the puncture of the subarachnoid space. The supraspinal ligament extends from one spinous process to the other, being firmly adherent to their tips with its attachment that can be transformed into fibrocartilage tissue and thereby interfere with the puncture. This ligament is a resistant fibrous cord that bridges the processes from the sixth or seventh cervical vertebrae to the sacrum, and continues ventrally as a thin interspinal ligament stretched between the adjoining bodies of the spinous processes.[12]

In the upper cervical region, the ligamentum nuchae attached to the external occipital protuberance represents the continuation of the supraspinal ligament. The ligamentum nuchae is felt as a resistance to the passage of the needle in the cisternal puncture.

The intervertebral foramina contain the spinal nerves. Their roof is formed by the inferior part of the posterior articular facet and, partially, by the anterior articular facet. The intervertebral foramina are located ventrally to the posterior intervertebral joints below each pedicle. They are situated between the transverse processes in the cervical region and, anterior to them, in the thoracic and lumbar regions. They are oval in shape, smaller in the cervical segments of the spine, larger in the thoracic, and even more so in the lumbar regions. Myelography can delineate the relationship under normal and pathologic conditions between the spinal nerves and intervertebral foramina, especially if combined with tomography.

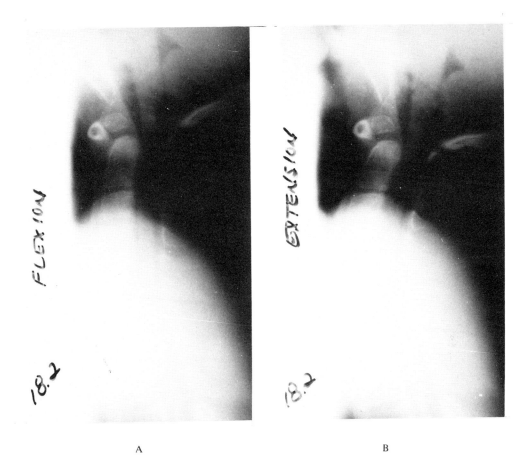

A   B

FIGURE 6. Ventrodorsal displacement of the spinal cord in flexion and extension of the neck on gas myelograms in the sagittal view of an infant.

II. THE RADIOLOGIC MEASUREMENTS

Physiologic displacements of the spinal cord in the canal can be easily established on gas myelography, with or without tomography (Figure 6). Regardless of the fact that the spinal cord is relatively fixed by the spinal nerves and the denticulate ligament, it will show the tendency to move ventrodorsally or dorsoventrally, depending upon the patient's position, that is, either supine, or prone.[13] The amplitudes or the movements can be measured on a series of lines drawn on tomograms after the subarachnoid space is first filled with oxygen. Each line connects the midpoint of the posterior surface of the vertebral bodies and of the odontoid with the corresponding point on the anterior surface of the vertebral arches. These lines form axes perpendicular to the longitudinal axis of the cord. Tomograms representing the sagittal midsection of the canal are used. Three to four such lines are drawn in the cervical region at the level of the first, second, fourth, and eventually sixth vertebrae. On each line, the width of the posterior longitudinal ligament of the epidural and anterior subarachnoid spaces, the spinal cord, and the posterior subarachnoid space is marked on two different tomograms, one with the spine in the supine position and the other with the spine in the prone (Figure 7).

These measurements carried out on 65 gas myelograms with no pathologic changes in the cervicodorsal area, have shown that the displacement of the cervical spinal cord

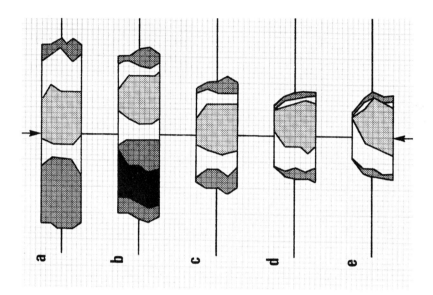

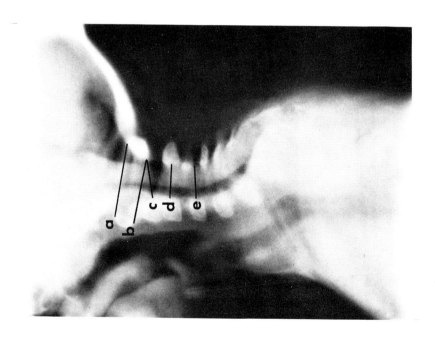

FIGURE 7.   Cervical area in the sagittal view with reference lines drawn on the gas myelogram. The number of lines can vary and they can also be used for the measurement of the thoracic region. In this 3-year-old girl, the measurement indicates a normal cervical spinal cord, as outlined on cross-sectional representations of each of the five levels on the polytomogram (see Volume II, Chapter 5, Section I).

varies from 2 to 5.5 mm. The same measurements have been applied in the dorsal and lumbar regions. The spinal cord shows less marked displacements in the thoracolumbar region. The cephalic and caudal enlargements of the spinal cord do not apparently interfere with its movements. Similar results have been obtained by Jirout.[14,15] The laminograms representing the midsection of the spinal canal filled with gas, with the patient lying on his lateral side, will show a less obvious lateral displacement of the spinal cord. On a series of tomograms obtained with polytome at a distance of 1 or 2 mm, the lateral displacement of the spinal cord has been 1 to 3.4 mm (Figure 1). The movements of the spinal cord in either direction are apparently more accentuated in children.

The length of the spinal cord measured on tomograms with the subarachnoid space filled with oxygen, has the tendency to vary according to the position of the spine. If the spine is in a marked anterior flexion, the conus will move 2 to 4 mm upwards. If the spine is in the maximal dorsal extension, it will move downwards about 2 to 3 mm.

Myelograms with positive or negative contrast media outline the shape of the spinal cord in the frontal projection (Figure 2). The shape of the spinal cord shows some variations related to the movements. Changes in shape and position of the spinal cord can be considerable in the presence of space occupying lesions in the spinal canal (see Chapter 10, Figure 13).

Movements of the cervical spinal cord will be reduced, or nonexisting, if the intracranial pressure is elevated.[14,15] In a marked tonsillar herniation due to intracranial hypertension, or in the Arnold-Chiari malformation, the cord is fixed in a ventral position, often slightly deviated to one side (see Chapter 8, Figure 2; Chapter 10, Figure 12). However, the increased intracranial pressure without tonsillar herniation can cause a dorsal displacement of the spinal cord, as described by Jirout.[15]

Deep inspiration, coughing, straining, or other modified Valsalva maneuvers will generally reduce the size of the subarachnoid space because of the increased filling of the epidural veins under these conditions. The column of the contrast material in the subarachnoid space will be displaced cranially, and it becomes narrower. On the other hand, a bilateral jugular compression will widen the column of the contrast in the subarachnoid sac due to the diminished filling of the epidural veins and the rise of pressure in the subarachnoid space. Equally, depending on the filling of the epidural venous plexus, tomograms will show a narrow epidural space in the upright position of the patient if compared with the horizontal.

It was assumed that the points of attachment of the denticular ligament to the dura mater prevented the movements of the spinal cord. Anatomic studies done by Breig[16] showed that the distance between the points of attachment of the denticular ligament depended upon the movements of the spine. If the canal is elongated as in the ventral flexion, the points of attachment diverge. In the lateral flexion of the spine, the attachments on the concave side converge. In addition, the studies done by Stoltmann and Blackwood[17] indicated that the denticulate ligament did not interfere, to a large extent, with the ventrodorsal movements of the cord, but it did affect its craniocaudal displacements.

Cinemyelography has contributed to the better understanding of the motions of the spinal cord.[18] Done with either positive or negative contrast media, cinemyelography shows that the denticulate ligament with its points of attachment follows the stretching or shrinking of the dura mater caused by the movements of the spinal canal. The denticulate ligament supports the spinal cord in its position in the spinal canal, yet it allows a certain degree of its movements. In injury to the spine, the denticulate ligament softens or prevents the direct transmission of the external acting force from the spinal wall to the cord, preserving, as much as possible, the width of the subdural space filled with CSF. The denticulate ligament follows the dura, or the spinal cord, or both, in the ventrodorsal or lateral extension and flexion of the spine, as well as in the prone or supine positions of the spine. The meningeal sheaths surrounding the spinal nerves in the foramina and the roots of these nerves fixed to the cord and the foramina, affect considerably more the mobility of the spinal cord. Cinemyelography done with positive or negative contrast media shows variations in the size and shape of the contrast column in the meningeal extensions around the spinal nerves. If the nerve roots are stretched, the contrast medium becomes very thin or vanishes from the sleeves. Dorsoventral or craniocaudal movements of the cord appear to be much more restricted by the spinal nerves and their meningeal sheaths fixed in the foramina and by the filum terminale, than by the action of the denticulate ligament.

Methods of radiologic measurements of the spinal cord play a significant role in the presence of the pathologic changes that have the tendency to either reduce or increase the size of the spinal cord. Different methods of radiologic measurement of the spinal cord and the surrounding spaces have been studied and applied with the intention to disclose, as early as possible, the presence of a disease. However, a radiologic determination of the size of the spinal cord differs from anatomopathologic methods since it is influenced by normal anatomic properties in patients, and by the physical factors that affect the radiographs.[19-22]

Magnification is one of the factors that intervenes with measurements of the spinal cord, in addition to geometric blurring, blurring due to the film and intensifying screens.[27] Sources of error can also be in the contrast medium, the measuring technique, and the observer.

The transverse diameter of the spinal cord can be established by means of positive contrast myelography through the use of a more penetrating technique. In the prone position, the insoluble contrast medium fills the ventral compartment of the subarachnoid space due to the specific gravity. The cord is encompassed by the lateral subarachnoid gutters filled with the contrast material. Any considerable enlargement involving the transverse diameter of the spinal cord can be recognized in this projection (Figure 8). On the basis of the measurements done in this position, Khilnani and Wolf have established a relationship between the width of the transverse diameter of the spinal cord and the width of the subarachnoid space that is not influenced by the magnification, and which represents a constant value with the normal average of 0.67.[25] Under normal conditions, the spinal cord occupies about ⅔ of the subarachnoid space. If this index or the cord-subarachnoid ratio is greater than 80% or less than 50%, it should be considered as abnormal.[26,28]

More subtle changes in the transverse diameter of the spinal cord may remain undetected in the prone position. If some doubts exist, the measurements should be done in the supine position. In the supine position, the contrast medium fills the posterior compartment of the subarachnoid space, and more so the lateral gutters. The cord is generally well outlined in the cervicodorsal region, especially if the lateral gutters are filled with the contrast gradually so that a narrow stream runs along the sides of the spinal cord.

Measurements of the transverse diameter done with insoluble contrast media are particularly valuable for the cervical region in the prone position, as well as for the cervicodorsal in the supine. An accurate determination of the sagittal diameter is more difficult to achieve even if the subarachnoid space is fully filled with an opaque insoluble contrast material.

If the anterior and the posterior compartments of the subarachnoid space are fully filled with gas, the shadow of the spinal cord stands out clearly between the ventral and dorsal radiolucent band of the gas. In this way, the sagittal diameter of the spinal cord becomes accessible to radiologic scrutiny. Gas myelography combined with polytomography offers a sharply delineated picture of the whole length of the spinal cord

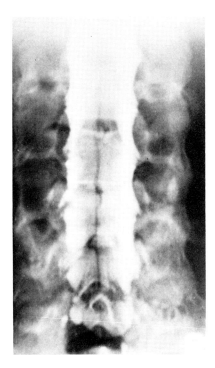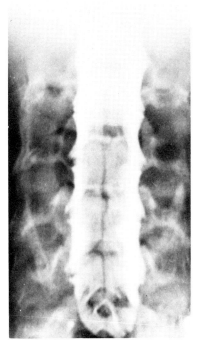

FIGURE 8.   Normal cervical myelogram clearly shows the anterior spinal artery and few tributaries. The spinal cord as seen is accessible to measurements in the anteroposterior view. The nerve roots are apparent emerging from the spinal cord and surrounded by meningeal sheaths at the level of foramina. Minor spondylotic spurs are also visible in the lower cervical region.

in its sagittal projection (Figure 9). The transverse diameter of the spinal cord in the supine position can be determined on gas myelolaminograms, in the lumbar and lower thoracic regions, if the physiologic curves of the spine are minimized by bending and raising the patient's legs (see Volume 2, Chapter 1, Figure 7). Yet, the curves of the cervical and upper dorsal areas cannot be reduced sufficiently. Gas myelolaminograms of these segments in the coronal plane will show only short portions of the cord. Therefore, a whole series of tomograms should be combined so that a complete outlining of the spinal cord is obtained. Obviously, this is not a method of choice to analyze the transverse diameter of the spinal cord in the cervical and upper thoracic regions. In this respect, positive contrast myelography has the priority.

Some pathologic processes in their initial phase may have more of an affect on the sagittal diameter of the spinal cord than the transverse (vascular diseases, long lasting compression, amyotrophic lateral sclerosis, syringomyelia, Friedreich's ataxia, tabes dorsalis, some intra- or extramedullary tumors, etc.). Consequently, gas myelography may prove to have some diagnostic advantages in these conditions. Actually, the atrophy of the spinal cord, regardless of its etiology, is reflected first in the reduction of the sagittal diameter of the cord (Figure 10). The possibility of recognizing this type of structural change of the cord is related to the feasibility of establishing the values of the normal sagittal diameter. Hence, a system of measurements of the sagittal diameter should be applied in order to estimate the alterations in the size of the spinal cord.

The study of the sagittal diameter of the spinal cord and the subarachnoid space, in

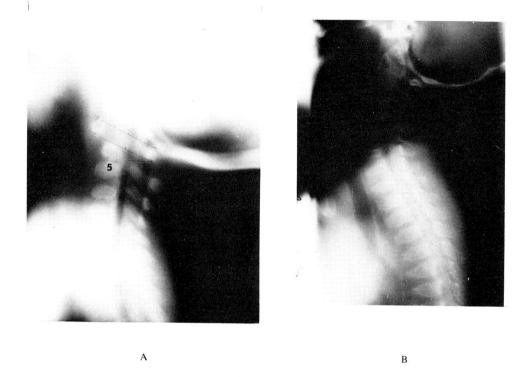

A   B

FIGURE 9(A). Gas myelogram of this 4-year-old boy outlines the cervical spinal cord and the lines drawn on it used as axes for the measurements of the sagittal diameter. (B) In infants, the whole length of the spinal cord can be presented on one polytomogram as seen here. In adults, three or four polytomograms are necessary to determine the length of the spinal cord and its sagittal diameters at different levels. Chapter 1 of Volume II deals more in detail with this matter.

different age groups, done by Nordquist, has clearly defined the dimensions of the sagittal diameter at different levels of the spinal cord. These measurements can be applied as a reliable guide in gas myelography.[23] Nordquist performed myelography on 101 autopsied cases. He carried out, mostly in sagittal projection, a series of measurements on myelograms from the first cervical to the first lumbar vertebra, and compared them to the values obtained by measuring the removed and the fixed spinal cord. Thereupon, the cases were divided into four age groups. The first group represented children from 0 to 10 years, the second included adults from 18 to 49 years (group A), the third consisted of adults from 50 to 69 years (group B), and the last one was the advanced age group from 70 to 88 years (C). In regard to the anatomic specimen of the cord, the effect of post-mortem swelling was estimated to be 2 to 4%. No significant changes in size could be found after the removal of the cord from the formalin solution, contrary to the observations of some other authors.[26] Comparing the values obtained from myelograms with those from spinal cord preparations, Nordquist found that differences exist especially in the cervical and lumbar regions. The position of the spine apparently does not influence the sagittal diameter of the cord according to the measurements on myelograms that he took in the supine, prone, lateral, and oblique positions. Diameters of the spinal cord and the subarachnoid space were measured on the lines drawn on myelograms, from the midpoint of the posterior surface of the vertebral body at right angles, to the longitudinal axis of the cord. According to Nordquist's observations, the sagittal diameter of the spinal cord already large at birth, increases rapidly thereupon, so that at the age of 9 it is about 0.65 mm smaller than in adults. Equally, the subarachnoid space at the age of 10, on the average, is 0.56

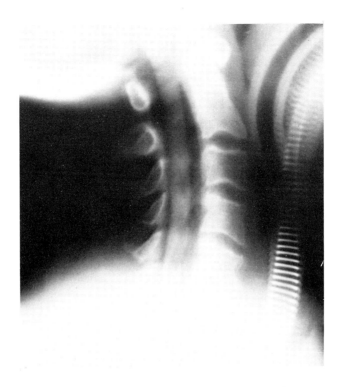

FIGURE 10. Atrophy of the spinal cord illustrated on this gas polytomogram resulted from the radiation therapy of the neck. The sagittal diameter is reduced by about 15%.

mm narrower than in adults. Furthermore, Nordquist concluded that the variations
between individuals are relatively considerable regarding the sagittal diameter of the
cord, and that the width of the subarachnoid space at different levels varies among
the three above-mentioned age groups.

The sagittal diameters indicate that the cervical enlargement of the spinal cord begins
between the second and the third cervical vertebrae, and its maximal width is at the
level of the fourth cervical vertebrae (mean value of 9.58 mm). The shortest sagittal
diameter of the thoracic spinal cord is between the fifth and the eighth dorsal vertebrae
(mean value of 7.39 mm). The lumbar enlargement begins about the tenth thoracic
vertebra. The mean values of the sagittal diameters are 8.40 mm at D_{11}, 9.62 mm at
D_{12}, and 9.95 mm at L_1 levels.

Taking into consideration all the factors that might affect radiologic evaluation of
the sagittal diameter of the spinal cord, Nordquist established tables for all age groups
that show mean values of the sagittal diameter at all levels, beginning with the second
cervical and ending with the first lumbar vertebrae. He could not recognize the differences in the width of the sagittal diameter between women and men. However, he
observed the changes in the size and shape of the cord in the advanced age, as well as
a decrease of the sagittal diameter of the subarachnoid space in the cervical region,
and an increase in the dorsal area (group C). Measurable physiologic atrophic changes
of the spinal cord were observed only after the age of 70. The reduction of the sagittal
diameter may also be influenced, to some extent, by the changes in the shape of the
cord at this age. Histologic studies revealed demyelination, hypertrophy of the pia
(recognizable macroscopically), proliferation of the interstitial connective tissue, senile
angiofibrosis, hyalin degeneration in the walls of the blood vessels, and hypertrophy

of the glia. These findings related to the spinal cord in advanced age are similar to the ones recorded by other authors.[29,30]

Jirout has also determined the width of the epidural and the subarachnoid spaces and of the spinal cord at different levels, on the basis of radiologic measurements taken on gas myelograms. The tables with the values calculated by Jirout speak once more in favor of eliminating the subjective factor as much as possible, and of introducing the objective methods of measurements of the spinal cord.[24] Other measurement techniques have been developed, also proving to be helpful in estimating the sagittal or transverse diameters of the contents of the spinal canal.[26,31-33]

Regardless of all the studies done in this field, the fact remains that the differences between the normal maximal and the normal minimal values of the diameters of the spinal cord are considerable. This is to say that if the sagittal or transverse diameters of the spinal cord in a patient are in the upper limits of the normal, an expansive intramedullary lesion can be present if the real diameters of his cord are in the lower limit of the determined values. On the other hand, if the spinal cord is undergoing a loss of substance (degeneration, atrophy), and the measurements are in the lower normal limits, the diagnosis can be missed if the real values are in the upper normal limits. Myelographic measurements would be more precise and informative if they could be established at the same time on the entire spinal cord in the coronar and sagittal projections of the patient. This possibility, most likely, depends upon the further development of adequate contrast media and techniques.

Some pathologic processes involving the spinal cord and the adjacent tissues in the canal can cause changes of the bony structures of the spine. Therefore, the established measurements of the spinal canal and the pedicles can be of further use in disclosing these intraspinal lesions.[7]

III. BLOOD SUPPLY OF THE SPINAL CORD

The arterial blood supply of the cord and the adjacent soft tissues has been the object of intensive studies since it was demonstrated that different lesions involving the spinal cord could be recognized by means of the spinal cord angiography. The introduction of this diagnostic technique makes possible the radiologic exploration of all medullary segments, and yields valuable information in vascular spinal malformations, medullary compression, and ischemia.

A thorough understanding of angiographic anatomy of the arterial distribution of the spinal cord is essential to the application and interpretation of angiography. The medullary arterial blood supply derives from several main sources which are the verterbral arteries, ascending cervical, intercostal, lumbar, iliolumbar, and lateral sacral arteries. An abundant network of arteries arises from these trunks, surrounds the cord, and extends into its inner substance. Thus the spinal cord is well vascularized, except for the midthoracic region, which has a rather poor blood supply.[10,34,35]

For the purposes of an angiographic diagnosis, the spinal cord arteries can be divided into two main groups, the outer or extramedullary, and the inner or intramedullary arteries. Although the outer arteries are linked by numerous anastomoses, and the inner ones derive from the outer, the spinal cord can be affected in different ways by the diseases of these vessels, and by a deficiency in their blood flow. The angiographic appearance of pathologic processes differs if they involve external or internal vessels. Furthermore, for the convenience of angiographic studies, the external group of arteries can be divided into longitudinal arteries that cover the whole length of the cord, and segmental arteries that reinforce the blood flow at certain levels.

Longitudinal arterial trunks are composed of the anterior and the two posterior spinal arteries. The anterior spinal artery extends from the foramen magnum to the filum terminale situated in the pia mater on the ventral surface of the spinal cord along the median fissure.[5,6] The two spinal arteries, the right and the left, ascend from the vertebral arteries above the posterior inferior cerebellar arteries and descend ventrally to the medulla oblongata to merge at the level of the foramen magnum and form the anterior spinal artery. These two vessels often vary in size and can be asymetric. Their junction with the upper segment of the anterior spinal artery appears on myelograms and angiograms in the characteristic shape of the letter Y (see Chapter 7, Figure 10). However, this pattern changes as a result of anatomic variations. In 25% of cases, the anterior spinal artery originates from multiple small arteries. The two anterior spinal arteries can be present in the cervical region. They generally fuse below their origin into one ventral arterial trunk.

Along its course, the anterior spinal artery sends off branches, the sulcal arteries, into the slit of the ventral median fissure, and supply with blood the membrane and the anterior halves of the spinal cord substance. The anterior spinal artery can have a tortuous appearance, mostly at the level of the spinal cord enlargements, or its course can be interrupted.[34] Its caliber may vary owing to its narrowness in the dorsal region. The arterial trunk assumes, occasionally, a beaded or segmented shape, being wider at the points of junction with the radiculomedullary arteries. The anterior spinal artery receives a supplementary blood flow from the two branches of the radioculomedullary arteries. The higher of these two branches is the smaller one, and the lower branch the larger. Thus, the anterior spinal artery can be considered as a segmented channel rather than a continuous arterial trunk, due to the inflow of blood from the ascending and descending branches originating from the radioculomedullary arteries at different levels.[36] About 1 cm above the tip of the conus medullaris, the anterior spinal artery forms an anastomotic arch with the two posterior spinal arteries. The anterior spinal artery ends following the filum terminale.

The two posterior or posterolateral spinal arteries emerge from the vertebral arteries at the level of medulla oblongata, actually, at the point of junction between the ascending branch of the second radicular artery and the posterior spinal branch of the vertebral artery. The posterior spinal arteries have an almost parallel course and a smaller caliber than the anterior spinal artery. Generally, they are well formed in the cervical and lumbar regions, but they can be discontinued quite often in the dorsal area. They pass dorsally to the medulla oblongata and descend longitudinally along the surface of the spinal cord, being situated ventrally to the posterior root of the spinal nerve. They are reinforced by the additional blood inflow from the ascending and descending branches of the posterior radiculomedullary arteries. The posterior spinal arteries end at the level of the conus medullaris forming the anastomotic arch with the anterior spinal artery known as the anastomotic arcade of the conus.[37]

The three spinal arteries together with the ascending and descending end branches of the radicular arteries form, around the spinal cord, three longitudinal arterial tracts that communicate within themselves by a rich network of obliquely or crosswise directed anastomoses. This arterial system is known as the perimedullary coronary arterial plexus (vasocorona perimedullaris.)[34]

The segmental arteries consist of the spinal rami that arise on both sides of the spine, entering the spinal canal through the intervertebral foramina, and divide at the corresponding segments into the anterior and posterior branch. These branches, called anterior and posterior spinal radicular arteries, follow the ventral and dorsal nerve roots towards the spinal cord, supplying the dura mater with blood. The anterior radicular arteries are situated in the anterior subarachnoid compartment, ventrally to the denticulate ligament, while the posterior are located in the posterior compartment and dorsally to the denticulate ligament. About 6 to 8 radicular arteries contribute to the anterior vascular system of the spinal cord, whereas 10 to 23 reinforce the posterior circulation of the cord. The origin, number, and course of the radicular arteries vary.[38] The radiculomedullary arteries divide into an ascending and a descending branch that anastomose with the upper and lower branch of the adjacent radiculomedullary arteries. The blood flow is directed cranially in the upper branch, and caudally in the lower one. Hence, variable ascending and descending blood flow currents can exist in the anterior and posterior spinal arteries. Angiography can demonstrate reversals of the blood flow in the anterior spinal artery in some pathologic conditions. It is possible that the changes in the direction of the blood flow can produce steal phenomena.[39,40]

On the basis of the segmented vascular architecture of the three longitudinal arterial tracts, Lazorthes has suggested a division of the blood supply to the spinal cord into three anatomic, physiologic, and functional territories: cervical, midthoracic, and dorsolumbar.[40] This division is convenient from the angiographic standpoint.

The cervical territory receives the blood supply from the vetebral arteries first through the two spinal arteries that form the anterior spinal artery, second, from a few lower branches out of which the most constant is the one following the third cervical nerve root. Lower, a prominent radicular artery derives from the deep cervical artery and accompanies the sixth cervical root (the artery of the cervical enlargement of Lazorthes). The next lower radicular artery originates from the costocervical trunk and runs along the eighth cervical nerve. From these vessels originate the radioculomedullary arteries which, in their course, meet the anterior and posterior spinal arteries. The size, number, and origin of the radicular arteries in the cervical region vary.[2,7] Nevertheless, the cervical region of the spinal cord receives an abundant blood supply from the radicular arteries, and the segments of the anterior and posterior spinal arteries have a considerable additional arterial inflow.

The region covered by the first seven thoracic vertebrae is referred to as the dorsal territory. The blood supply to this area is relatively poor. A radicular artery, often unilateral, follows the fourth or the fifth nerve and provides the anterior spinal artery with radiculomedullary branches. The additional segmental blood supply to the posterior spinal arteries is just as poor.[10] In the dorsal territory, angiography can often disclose the interruptions of the anterior or posterior spinal arteries that further decrease the blood flow in this region.

Below the eighth thoracic vertebra begins the dorsolumbar territory. The main segmental contributor in this area is the arteria radicularis anterior magna described by Adamkiewicz.[41,42] This is a major, usually single artery, originating on the left side mostly (80%), which is particularly important for the angiographic technique. In most instances, it enters the spinal canal following one of the spinal nerve roots between the ninth thoracic and second lumbar vertebrae (85%). However, occasionally (15%), this vessel may have a high location between the fifth and the eighth thoracic vertebrae.

The artery of Adamkiewicz has a rather long course, and often branches at the anterior median sulcus into an ascending as well as into a wider descending vessel, about the level of the tenth thoracic vertebra. The descending branch, situated anteriorly to the ventral median fissure, continues downwards thus joining the anastomotic arch of the conus. On angiograms, the upper part of the artery of Adamkiewicz may have a hairpin-like shape. The ascending direction of this artery can be explained by the embryologic disproportion in the growth of the spinal cord and the spine.[36] A posterior radiculomedullary branch can arise, in addition, from the artery of Adamkiewicz.[43] The significance of this vessel is disputed.

The lumbar, ileolumbar, and sacral arteries produce branches that accompany the nerve roots of the cauda equina. In case of circulatory insufficiency in the lower segment of the spinal cord, these vessels may become wider and can reinforce the blood supply of the lower part of the cord.[44]

The segmental distribution of the blood flow and its ramification into the three territories of the spinal cord require a more complex angiographic technique in order to visualize the whole system of the blood circulation. An adequate technique of injection of the contrast medium into all major feeding branches becomes even more important if the anterior or posterior spinal arteries have a normally interrupted course, or their width changed.

A collateral circulation can provide the blood flow for the upper cervical spinal cord if a circulatory insufficiency develops in the vertebral or subclavian arteries. The arterial blood can reach the cord through the branches of the inferior posterior cerebellar arteries, the muscular branches of the vertebral arteries, the ascending cervical, or occipital arteries. The lower segment of the cervical spinal cord can be supplied with blood by the branches of the superior and inferior thyroid arteries, internal mammary arteries, vertebral arteries, and the deep or ascending cervical arteries. The anastomotic arch of the conus medullaris provides collateral circulation for the dorsolumbar area. The anterior and posterior lumbosacral radicular arteries contribute as well to the arterial perfusion of the conus in case of an arterial obstruction.[45,46]

The inner vascular supply of the spinal cord arises mainly from the sulcal arteries and the vasocorona perimedullaris. Sulcal or central intraspinal perforating branches are directed radially, bringing the blood to both sides of the spinal cord, which are separated by the ventral median fissure. They arise from the anterior spinal artery, being densely distributed at the levels of the cervical and the lumbar enlargements, and more scarcely in the thoracic area. Their ramifications in the substance of the spinal cord provide the arterial blood flow in the pyramidal and spinothalamic (Edinger) tracts, to the fasciculus gracilis (Goll), the fasciculus cuneatus (Burdach), the anterior columns of the gray substance, the area of the gray comissure, the ventral part of the dorsal gray columns, and to the dorsal nucleus (Clark's column). These arterial branches meet those deriving from the vasocorona and cover a large, functionally important part of the intramedullary structures in the white and gray substances.

Arteries originating from the vascorona perimedullaris radiate into the substance of the cord, supplying, with their shorter or longer branches, mainly the posterior columns of the gray matter, the dorsal aspect of the gray comissure, the lateral and dorsal funiculus, and the posterior septum.[35]

The venous system of the spinal canal consists of an external plexus around the spine, an internal plexus within the spinal canal situated between the dura and the wall of the canal, the basivertebral and intervertebral veins, and the spinal cord veins. Some lesions invading different components of the spinal canal can be recognized on phlebograms done by filling these venous systems with a contrast agent.

The external vertebral venous system surrounding the spine is formed by an anterior and posterior plexus connected with multiple venous anastomoses. The intervertebral and basivertebral veins meet the anterior external plexus. The internal vertebral venous plexus includes longitudinal veins situated anteriorly and posteriorly between the bony structures, disks, and ligaments on one side, and the dura mater on the other. The two anterior veins, one on each side of the posterior longitudinal ligament, are connected to the basivertebral veins with the posterior internal vein communicating with the posterior external plexus. The anterior and posterior internal venous systems are linked by a network of ring-like anastomoses.

The veins of the spinal cord form in the pia mater a plexus around the cord. Two more prominent, longitudinal veins can be recognized. The larger one is located posteriorly to the dorsal median sulcus and the anterior ventrally to the anterior median fissure. Moreover, about four smaller veins are present posterior to the spinal nerve roots and lateral to the spinal cord which they follow in a longitudinal way. The radiculomedullary veins drain this venous plexus or venous vasocorona. They do not necessarily accompany the arteries, and their size, position, and number vary. However, in the lower thoracic region, a vena radiculomedullaris is usually present, located mostly on the left dorsal side of the spinal cord.

Intramedullary veins emerge from the substance of the spinal cord to join the venous vasocorona at different points. Along the anterior median fissure and the posterior median sulcus, the anterior and posterior median veins leave the spinal cord. Some veins appear from the cord along the nerve roots, whereas others arise among the veins forming the anastomotic chain around the spinal cord.[47,48] In the upper cervical region, the venous system around the cord fuses into several small venous channels that communicate with the vertebral veins, and drain into the inferior petrosal sinuses or into the inferior cerebellar veins.

Different venous plexuses of the spine are linked together by means of multiple anastomotic channels. The external vertebral plexus meets in the lumbar region the ascending lumbar vein. In the thoracic area, it drains into the azygos and hemiazygos veins, and in the cervical region it flows into the superior intercostal and azygos veins.[2,14] Phlebographies done by Batson have shown the variety of possible communications between the veins of the spine and the major systemic venous channels.[49]

IV. THE CSF

The CSF fills the subarachnoid space with its various cisterns, the central canal of the spinal cord, and the ventricles. It is discharged either by the tortuous thin-walled vessels of the choroid plexus under hydrostatic pressure, or by the secretion of the epithelial cells that cover the vessels of the plexus, or by the combination of the two mechanisms. The CSF is mostly discharged by the choroid plexuses located in the lateral, the third, and fourth ventricles. There is also evidence that a smaller quantity of the CSF is produced by the ependymal secretion in the central spinal canal and by the nervous tissue. Among its different probable functions, one is purely mechanical. It protects the CNS, including the spinal cord and its nerves, from an external acting force. The CSF is interposed as an elastic cushion between the spinal cord and the external wall of the spine. In addition, it has an effect on the intracranial pressure, and according to more recent studies, it takes part in the metabolism of the CNS.[50,51] Some of the properties of the CSF are of special significance to the performance of different types of myelographies, which will be discussed later.[52,54]

The CSF runs from the lateral ventricles to the fourth ventricle. In the fourth ventricle, some fluid emerging from the central canal of the cord is added to the fluid formed by the plexuses. The CSF leaves the ventricles through the foramina of Luschka and the foramen of Magendie and fills the subarachnoid space. The subarachnoid space extends around the vessels into the nervous tissue and forms the perivascular spaces that further divide according to the ramifications of the vessels. They end at the point of fusion of the pia mater and the arachnoid. The metabolic products and inflammatory exudates with cells probably reach the CSF by means of the perivascular spaces. It is possible that the CSF is augmented by an inflow from the perivascular spaces and from the lymphatics of the peripheral and cranial nerves.[10]

The CSF flows first down around the spinal cord, then its stream diverts cranially towards the base of the brain and the convexity of the hemispheres, where through the arachnoid villi it drains into the venous system of the sagittal sinus and its lacunae. The study done by Welch and Friedman indicates that the arachnoid villi may act as valves. If the pressure of the CSF rises, they will open and drain the fluid.[53] A small

of Thorotrast® for diagnostic purposes was expressed in numerous papers that appeared after its introduction in 1928.[33,35-37]

Moniz et al. used Thorotrast® as a contrast medium for cerebral angiography.[33] After the exposure and puncture of the carotid artery, Moniz injected about 8 to 10 cc of Thorotrast® into the circulation and obtained very good angiographies on a seriograph known as "radio-carrousel" (constructed by Caldas). Moniz concluded his study, published in 1933, stating that he preferred Thorotrast® (manufactured by Heyden in Dresden) to the solution of iodide (25% sodium iodide, Abrodil®) for cerebral angiography, and believed that it was the substance of choice for this procedure.[34]

Radovici and Meller, in 1932, were the first to report upon the application of Thorotrast® in the exploration of subarachnoid spaces.[35] In their publication, Radovici and Meller described their experimental work with colloidal thorium (Umbrathor®) and the first myelography carried out in a paralytic patient with 5 cc of Thorotrast®.[35]

The extensive use of Thorotrast® for different diagnostic procedures was to some extent changed owing to the appearance of publications pointing to the disadvantages of this compound. Thus, a controversial attitude towards Thorotrast® became apparent. In reviewing the initial publications concerning clinical application of Thorotrast®, it is rather surprising to find that the question of its radioactivity had been ignored, and mentioned in some articles as something remotely possible and probably inconsequential.[32,33,35-37] This neglect of radioactive capabilities of thorium is especially astonishing bearing in mind that some excellent studies dealing with this problem had been published earlier. For example, Martland, in his two articles concerning occupational poisoning in workers who were employed in manufacturing luminous watch dials, clearly documented the complications that could occur as a result of the radioactive nature of thorium.[39,40] The detailed work of Martland disclosed the destructive power of alpha particles on workers who, by pointing brushes repeatedly in their mouths, swallowed the paint that consisted of crystalline phosphorescent zinc sulphite, rendered luminous by the addition of radium mesothorium and radiothorium.[39,40]

It became rather conspicuous that the elimination of Thorotrast® from the body was insignificant and that thorium dioxide remained attached in the reticulo-endothelial system, especially in the spleen and liver, practically indefinitely.[41-45,55] In addition, over periods of months, most investigators confirmed a stable radioactivity of thorium in different organs.[43,51] The more they became apparent, undesirable effects of Thorotrast® were extensively documented and stirred an unfavorable reaction regarding the usage of this contrast medium.[42] As an example, in 1932, the Council on Pharmacy and Chemistry of the American Medical Association advised the discontinuation of the intravenous application of Thorotrast® for radiologic visualization of the liver and spleen.[47]

Histological changes of the nervous system that occurred after the introduction of Thorotrast® into the subarachnoid spaces were mentioned by Radovici and Meller (1932).[35] The comprehensive review of the clinical and experimental results with Thorotrast® by Reeves and Stuck in 1938, and later, the detailed study of Hughs in 1953, depict clearly the deleterious action of this contrast medium on the CNS and other tissues.[42,44] Beres confirmed the extensive damage consisting of desquamation of the ependymal lining and macrophagic accumulations in the ventricular cavities, around the choroid plexus, and in the subarachnoid spaces.[48] Macrophages containing Thorotrast® were found in the perivascular spaces of the subependymal areas. Well documented experimental and clinical studies proved that thorium could cause the development of sarcoma, carcinoma, and fibroma in different tissues.[49,50,54,55]

Although Thorotrast® had good properties as a radiopaque contrast medium, it

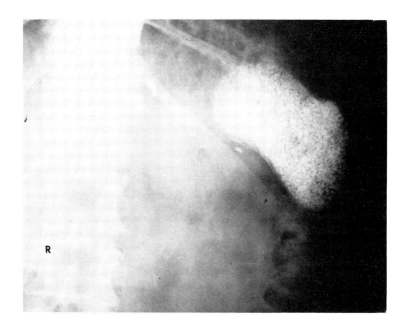

FIGURE 1.   Radiograph of the abdomen of this 82-year-old female patient obtained in the course of the radiologic examination of her stomach revealed a dense opacification of the spleen and partially of the liver. The patient had had an angiography performed with Thorotrast® about 40 years earlier.

had to be abandoned to the regret of many users for its emanation of alpha "rays" that were more destructive than either the beta or gamma rays if localized permanently within a tissue.[38,39,43,46,51,52] Furthermore, the toxic and mechanical effect of Thorotrast® on the cells could not be eliminated. Some authors noted an extreme lymphatic destruction after injections of Thorotrast®, and they speculated enthusiastically upon the use of this material in a metastatic invasion of lymph nodes as a curative procedure.[53] Owing to its permanent attachment to the tissues, even today, we can find radiographs of the spleen or liver, or other areas of the body partially or completely filled with Thorotrast® that was injected many years ago. In recent literature, we can find articles and studies dealing with the problems related to the effects of Thorotrast® used up to 40 or more years previously.[55,57] The application of Thorotrast® was more or less abandoned in the early Forties after clear evidence had been established about its unfavorable effects.[42,48,54,56] In 1938 Nosik introduced his forced drainage technique intended to remove Thorotrast® from the subarachnoid space after myelography, assuming that this procedure might eliminate the noxious effects[58] (Figure 1).

The search for a less harmful compound that could be used in the exploration of subarachnoid space continued. In 1942 Lefft, among other researchers, introduced his diiodotyrosine-gelatin contrast medium (Tyrogel®).Diiodotyrosine is an amino acid containing 58% of iodine by molecular weight.[59] It is an intermediary product of thyroxine, normally found in the thyroid gland. The diiodotyrosine in gelatin proved to be miscible with the spinal fluid and quite radiopaque. The gelatin had the capability to hold the diiodotyrosine in suspension in the spinal fluid, long enough to provide the necessary time for the performance of the radiologic examination. As diiodotyrosine in gelatin was heavier than the spinal fluid, it gravitated to the lower portion of the spinal canal or ventricles within a few hours after the injection. The absorption of this compound occurred after the breakdown of suspension.[59] Nonetheless, Tyrogel®️ caused rather severe reactions of the CNS, and thus its application became limited and of short duration.

Iodinated organic compounds (iodinated aracyl esters) were studied by Strain et al. at the University of Rochester, (New York) with the intention of developing an absorbable and insoluble fluid contrast medium for radiologic diagnostic purposes.[60] In their first report in 1942, they summarized the achieved results of this research work by stating that ethyl iodophenylundecylate, a mixture of isomers obtained by the addition of iodobenzene to ethyl undecylenate in the presence of aluminum chloride, appeared to meet most of the clinical requirements for a contrast medium.[60]

The next article by Plati et al. on iodinated organic compounds described in detail the experimental work preceding the introduction of ethyl iodophenylundecylate in 1943.[61] The third publication by Steinhausen et al. that appeared in 1944 dealt with the application of ethyl iodophenylundecylate as a contrast medium for intrathecal injections.[62] Thus, a new radiopaque agent was introduced for radiologic diagnostic procedures to be known as Pantopaque®️ "a name coined to provide the users with a convenient designation".[62] Before its clinical use, Pantopaque®️ was tested intrathecally in dogs and compared to the iodized poppy-seed oil. According to these authors, the new medium proved to be well tolerated by the experimental animals, and apparently completely absorbed within a year from the subarachnoid space. The iodized poppyseed oil, in their experience, was 22 times as viscous as ethyl iodophenylundecylate at 25°C, and 17 times as viscous at 37.5°C. The dogs used for the experiments had a short period of increased body temperature after the injection of 3 to 5 cc of Pantopaque®️. Sections taken from the spinal cord of dogs, sacrificed at different intervals, showed that Lipiodol®️ as well as Pantopaque®️ were encysted after approximately 6 weeks. Cord sections, after intrathecal injection of ethyl iodophenylundecylate, showed physiologic response around the cysts similar to the effects of foreign bodies. Steinhausen and co-workers speculated that this more rapid rate of absorption of the new medium might be the cause of a relatively greater toxicity, namely, intravenous injections in dogs showed that Pantopaque®️ was without effect at the level of 0.5 g/kg, but lethal at the level of 1.0 g/kg. Apparently, emulsification with water containing a small amount of Igepon-T®️ (sodium olelylmethyltaurine) or of methyl cellulose reduced the toxicity. Steinhausen and co-workers applied Pantopaque®️ in myelography for the first time on November 23, 1940 and from thereon, it has been tested and used extensively in different institutions.[62] In this third article, the authors, however, indicated the necessity of removal of the contrast medium from the subarachnoid space, using the procedure described by Kubik and Hampton.[29] They presumed that with this procedure, about 90% of the injected contrast medium could be easily removed and the small remaining amount would be absorbed in a few weeks. The fourth article in this series, published by Ramsey et al. in 1944, presented the first clinical review of 150 Pantopaque®️ myelograms.[63] The authors emphasized the fluidity of the new medium as an asset that simplified the myelographic procedure and the demonstration of smaller defects of the subarachnoid space that could not be detected with iodized poppy-seed oil. They gave a detailed description of the injection technique of 3 to 5 cc of Pantopaque®️ into the subarachnoid space, of fluoroscopic and radiographic techniques, and of the removal of Pantopaque®️.[63] In this fourth publication, the earlier mentioned necessity to remove Pantopaque®️ was reemphasized. The article concludes that the results in 150 cases of Pantopaque®️ myelographies show that the use of the new medium simplifies the procedure and leads to a higher diagnostic accuracy.[63] These four articles published in 1942, 1943, and 1944, introduced Pantopaque®️ into the radiologic practice as the most convenient for technical purposes and least toxic oily contrast medium for myelography. Since that period, up to the present date, Pantopaque® has been used for myelography and ventriculography in the majority of radiologic institutions, along with similar compounds introduced (in other countries) under different names (Myodil®, Éthiodol®, etc.)[69,79]

Camp, in his elaborate study related to myelography, mentioned that Pantopaque® was promptly accepted as a replacement for Lipiodol® and Thorotrast®.[64] However, he indicated that the rate of its absorption from the subarachnoid space was slow and since it was an oily medium, removal after the examination became necessary in order to avoid the same complications that were related to the retained Lipiodol®. Encysted collections of both substances have been found subsequent to myelography, and, in essence, the difference between the two media is largely a matter of viscosity. Since Pantopaque® and similar compounds are less viscous, and thus easier to aspirate, it has become the medium of choice for myelography. Even so, in Camp's experience, Lipiodol® had given more accurate information than Pantopaque,® especially concerning the lesions in the thoracic area of the spinal canal. He thought that Pantopaque® gave satisfactory information for the exploration of the lumbar and cervical regions, but because of its fluidity and increased rate of flow, complete filling of any desired level in the thoracic vertebral canal was difficult to obtain unless large amounts, such as 10 to 20 cc, were injected.[64]

The amount of Pantopaque® to be injected into the subarachnoid space became a matter of discussion that has been going on practically since its introduction into radiologic practice. Some recommended the use of smaller quantities, about 3 to 5 cc, and leaving Pantopaque® in the subarachnoid space after myelographic procedure was terminated. It was believed that such small amounts would not produce serious damage to the meninges or nerve roots and that they would be eventually resorbed.[78] Others, however, thought that a larger amount of contrast medium was necessary to clearly visualize the spinal subarachnoid space, and that an attempt should be made to remove the contrast medium after the examination.[64] More often, the so-called double contrast technique was applied, and Camp emphasized that the combination of gas and Pantopaque® was exceedingly helpful in the study of patients who had had previous laminectomies.[64] With an extensive and further utilization of Pantopaque®, it became more evident that this opaque medium could be the cause of meningismus, severe arachnoiditis, elevation of the number of cells, and protein in the CSF.[65-68] These and other possible complications, as well as the difficulty of removing Pantopaque® from the subarachnoid space, led to a more cautious approach in its usage, or to its complete elimination in some radiologic institutions.[70-72] It was obvious, however, that Pantopaque® or similar compounds were less noxious than Thorotrast® and more suitable for myelography than Lipiodol®, except for the more recent types of extra fluid Lipiodol® or Éthiodol® (ethyl ester of iodinated fatty acid of poppy-seed oil prepared with lecithin — 37% iodine).

In a similar way as with Lipiodol®, attempts were made to dilute Pantopaque® which, due to its relatively high content of iodine (30.5% by weight), was radiopaque to such an extent as to possibly mask an intraspinal, smaller, expansive lesion. This revival of experiments with more diluted Pantopaque® and similar compounds used as contrast media was described by different authors and more recently by Kieffer and co-workers.[73] The first diluted Pantopaque® had 15% of iodine by weight. Because of its relatively low specific gravity, this diluted contrast material flowed slowly in the subarachnoid space and caused considerable lengthening of myelographic procedure. Hence, a 22% concentration of iodine with specific gravity of 1.174 was introduced as a substitute for the standard Pantopaque®. This diluted Pantopaque® proved to be more convenient for usage than the 15% concentration. The breakdown into the small droplets as seen with standard Pantopaque® did not occur to the same degree with 15% dilution. To some extent, this cohesive characteristic of the contrast medium was retained with 22% dilution. It appears that larger volumes of diluted Pantopaque® were necessary in order to outline the entire subarachnoid space using the so-called full column technique. About 20 to 40 cc of 15 or 22% Pantopaque® were generally used, and in one instance Kieffer injected 105 cc. The increased incidence of side reactions with more diluted forms of Pantopaque®, as well as different technical difficulties, influenced the discontinuation of the use of these compounds.[73]

A renewed interest in the heavy metals occurred in the early Fifties and will be mentioned here for chronologic reasons. Since 1896 up to 1928, almost all elements with higher atomic weight in different chemical compounds have been analyzed, and some used experimentally as potential contrast media for hollow organs.[32] Mostly because of the toxicity that metal ions exert on tissues, the extensive experiments carried out with different elements were unsuccessful. In the 1950s, a type of metal-binding agent had opened a new avenue in this field. The metal chelating agent ethylenediaminetetraacetic acid (EDTA) drew special interest because various EDTA chelations apparently caused a decrease in toxicity of a number of metals as demonstrated by some experimental works.[74] However, this type of contrast media used in laboratories could not find its clinical implementation.[75,77]

In the 1960s, considerable attention was paid to crystalline suspension of B-(3-dimethylaminomethylinamino-2-4,6-triiodophenyl) propionic acid ethyl ester in the isotonic 5.5% glucose solution (61.45% iodine) known as SH 617 L. This compound, in the beginning, appeared quite attractive for its relatively fast absorption. However, being the cause of meningeal reactions with irritative and toxic effects, its clinical use was restricted.[75,76,78]

REFERENCES

1. Wustmann, O., Experimentelle Untersuchungen über die Relief-darstellung (Umrisszichung) des Zentralnerven systems in Röentgenbild durch Thoriumkontrast-Mittel, *Dtsch. Z. Chir.*, 238, 529, 1933.
2. Reeves, D. L. and Stuck, R. M., Clinical and experimental results with Thorotrast, *Medicine (Baltimore)*, 17, 37, 1938.
3. Belenger, J., Simons, M., Jeanmart, L., and Danis, A., Evolution de la Myelographie, *J. Belge Radiol.*, 54, 347, 1971.
4. Dandy, W. E., Ventriculography, *Ann. Surg.*, 68, 5, 1918.
5. Dandy, W. E., Experimental hydrocephalus, *Ann. Surg.*, 70, 129, 1919.
6. Sicard, J. A. and Forestier, J., Méthode générale d' exploration radiologique par l'huile iodée, *Bull. Memoires Soc. Med. Paris*, 46, 463, 1922.
7. Sicard, J. A. and Forestier, J., Injections intravasculaires d'huile iodée sous controle radiogique, *Compt. Rendu Soc. Biol. Paris*, 88, 1200, 1923.
8. Sicard, J. A. and LaPlane, L., Diagnostic des tumeurs rachidiennes forme pseudo-pottique; radiolipiodol, *Presse Med.*, 1, 33, 1925.
9. Forestier, J., Iodized oil (Lipiodol) in Roentgenology, *Am. J. Roentgenol.*, 15, 352, 1926.
10. Sicard, J. A. and Forestier, J., Roentgenologic exploration of the central nervous system with iodized oil (Lipiodol), *Arch. Neurol. Psychiatry*, 16, 420, 1926.
11. Sicard, J. A. and Forestier, J., *The Use of Lipiodol in Diagnosis*, Oxford University Press, London, 1932.
12. Ebaugh, F. G. and Mella, H., Use of Lipiodol in localization of spinal lesions, *Am. J. Med. Sci.*, 172, 117, 1926.
13. Peper, H., Die Myelographie in Dienste der Diagnostik von Erkrankungen des Rückenmarks, *Ergeb. Med. Strahlenforsch.*, 2, 107, 1926.
14. Albrecht, K., Die röntgenologische Darstellung von Rückenmarkstumoren Durch Jodipin, *Zentralbl. F. D. Ges. Neurol. u. Psychiat.*, 41, 921, 1925.
15. Wartenberg, R., Beitrag zur Encephalographie und Myelographie, *Arch. f. Psychiat.*, 77, 507, 1926.

16. Mixter, W. J. and Ayer, J. B., Radiography following the injection of iodipin into the spinal subarachnoid space, *Arch. Neurol. Psychiatry*, 11, 499, 1924.

17. Mixter, W. J., The use of Lipiodol in tumor of the spinal cord, *Arch. Neurol. Psychiatry*, 14, 35, 1925.

18. Mixter, W. J. and Barr, J. S., Rupture of the intervertebral disc with involvement of the spinal cord, *N. Engl. J. Med.*, 211, 210, 1934.

19. Hampton, A. O. and Robinson, J. M., Roentgenographic demonstration of rupture of the intervertebral disc into the spinal canal after the injection of Lipiodol; with special reference to unilateral lumbar lesions accompanied by low back pain with "sciatic" radiation, *Am. J. Roentgenol.*, 36, 782, 1936.

20. Lindblom, A. F., Effect of Lipiodol on meninges, *Acta Radiol. (Diagn. Stockholm)*, 5, 129, 1926.

21. Lindblom, A. F., On the effects of various iodized oils on the meninges, *Acta Med. Scand.*, 76, 395, 1931.

22. Bruskin, J. and Propper, N., Experimentelle Myelo-Encephalographie an Huden ünd uber den Einfluss von Iodipin und Lipiojodol auf das Rückenmark, Gerhirn und Dessen Haute, *Z. Gesamte Exper. Med.*, 75, 34, 1931.

23. Brown, H. A. and Carr, J. L., The effect of Lipiodol in the subarachnoid space, *Surg. Gynecol. Obstet.*, 68, 945, 1939.

24. Davis, L., Haven, H. A., and Stone, T. T., The effect of injections of iodized oil in the spinal subarachnoid space, *JAMA*, 94, 772, 1930.

25. Odin, M., Runström, G., and Lindblom, A. F., Iodized oils an aid to the diagnosis of lesions of the spinal cord and a contribution to the knowledge of adhesive circumscribed meningitis, *Acta Radiol. (Diagn. Stockholm)*, Suppl., 7, 1, 1928.

26. Craig, W. McK., The use and abuse of iodized oil in the diagnosis of lesions of the spinal cord, *Surg. Gynec. Obstet.*, 49, 17, 1929.

27. Marcovich, A. W., Walker, A. E., and Jessico, C. M., The immediate and late effects of the intrathecal injection of iodized oil, *JAMA*, 116, 2247, 1941.

28. Epstein, E. S., *The Spine*, 4th ed., Lea & Febiger, Philadelphia, 1976, 86.

29. Kubik, C. S. and Hampton, A. O., Removal of iodized oil by lumbar puncture, *N. Engl. J. Med.*, 224, 455, 1941.

30. Jaeger, R. Irritating effect of iodized vegetable oils on the brain and spinal cord when divided into small particles, *Arch. Neurol. Psychiatry*, 64, 715, 1950.

31. Arnell, S., Encephalography with solution of contrast-salt, *Acta Radiol. (Diagn. Stockholm)*, 13, 43, 1932.

32. Blühbaum, Th., Frik, K., and Kalkbrenner, H., Eine neue Anwendungsart der Kolloide in der Röntgendiagnostik. 1. Metteilung, *Fortschr. Röntgenstr.*, 37, 18, 1928.

33. Moniz, E., Pinto, A., and Lima, A., Le thorotrast dans l'encephalographie artérielle, *Rev. Neurol.*, 2, 646, 1931.

34. Moniz, E., Cerebral angiography with thorotrast, *Arch. Neurol. Psychiatry*, 29, 1318, 1933.

35. Radovici, A. and Meller, O., Essai de liquidographie cephalo-rachidienne. Encephalo-myelographie par le thorotrast sous-arachnoidien, *Bull. Acad. Med. Paris*, 107, 314, 1932.

36. Freeman, W., Schoenfeld, H. H., and Moore, C., Ventriculography with colloidal thorium dioxide, *JAMA*, 106, 96, 1936.

37. Veal, R. J. and McFetridge, E. M., Technical considerations in arteriography of the extremities with thorotrast, *Am. J. Roentgend.*, 32, 64, 1934.

38. Alexander, L., Jung, T. S., and Lyman, R. S., Colloidal thorium dioxide: its use in intracranial diagnosis and its fate on direct injection into the brain and the ventricles, *Arch. Neurol. Psychiatry*, 32, 1143, 1939.

39. Martland, H. S., Occupational poisoning in manufacture of luminous watch dials, *JAMA*, 92, 466, 1929.

40. Martland, H. S., Occupational poisoning in manufacture of luminous watch dials, *JAMA*, 92, 552, 1929.

41. Cooke, H. H., Hepatolienography; experimental study of the elimination of the contrast medium, *Arch. Surg. (Chicago)*, 29, 29, 1934.

42. Reeves, D. L. and Stuck, R. M., Clinical and experimental results with thorotrast, *Medicine*, 17, 37, 1938.

43. Jacobson, L. E. and Rosenbaum, D., Postmortem findings and radioactivity determinations five years after injection of thorotrast, *Radiology*, 31, 601, 1938.

44. Hughs, R. Chronic changes in the central nervous system following thorotrast ventriculography, *Proc. R. Soc. Med.*, 46, 191, 1953.

45. Ziffren, S. E., Accidental perivascular injection of thorotrast, *Radiology*, 34, 171, 1940.

46. **Weber, H. M. and Pugh, D. G.**, The present status of contrast myelography, *Am. J. Med. Sci.*, 206, 687, 1943.
47. Report of the Council on Pharmacy and Chemistry: Thorotrast, *JAMA*, 99, 2183, 1932.
48. **Beres, D.**, Effects of thorotrast (colloidal thorium dioxide) on ependymal lining and related parts of the brain, *Arch. Pathol. Lab. Med.*, 28, 49, 1939.
49. **McMahon, E. H., Murphy, A. S., and Bates, M. T.**, Endothelial-cell sarcoma of liver following thorotrast injections, *Am. J. Pathol.*, 23, 585, 1947.
50. **Fleming, A. J. and Chase, W. H.**, The effects of administration of thorium dioxide, *Surg. Gynecol. Obstet.*, 63, 145, 1936.
51. **Taft, R. B.**, Demonstration of gamma radiation from living patient following thorotrast injection, *Radiology*, 11, 530, 1937.
52. **Twining, E. W. and Rowbotham, C. F.**, Ventriculography by opaque injection, *Lancet*, 11, 122, 1935.
53. **Menville, L. J. and Ane, J. N.**, Roentgen visualization of lymph nodes in animals, *JAMA*, 98, 1796, 1932.
54. **Batzenschlager, A., Weill-Bousson, M., and Mandard, A. M.**, Cancers, Hépatique et biliaire par thorotrastose hépato-ganglionnaire, *Arch. Anat. Pathol.*, 15, 295, 1967.
55. **Roujeau, J., Caulin, C., Bescol-Liversac, J., Leclerc, J. P., Cornu, P., Lamy, Ph., Dentan, M., and Barbezat, S.**, Thorotrastose Hépato-Splénoganglionnaire, *Sem. Hôp. Paris*, 47, 818, 1971.
56. **Epstein, B. S.**, *The Spine*, 4th ed., Lea & Febiger, Philadelphia, 1976, 87.
57. **diChiro, G. and Fisher, R. L.**, Contrast radiography of the spinal cord, *Arch. Neurol. Chicago*, 11, 125, 1964.
58. **Nosik, W. A.**, Clinical application of thorotrast myelography and subsequent forced drainage. Report of a case, *Cleveland Clin. Q.*, 5, 262, 1938.
59. **Lefft, H. H. and MacLean, A. J.**, Visualization of the brain and spinal cord with diiodotyrosine-gelatin contrast medium, including observations on the fate of this material, *Arch. Neurol. Psychiatry*, 48, 843, 1942.
60. **Strain, W. H., Plati, J. T., and Warren, S. L.**, Iodinated organic compounds as contrast media for radiographic diagnoses. I. Iodinated aracyl esters, *J. Am. Chem. Soc.*, 64, 1436, 1942.
61. **Plati, J. T., Strain, W. H., and Warren, S. L.**, Iodinated organic compounds as contrast media for radiographic diagnoses. II. Ethyl esters of iodinated straight and branched chain phenyl fatty acids, *J. Am. Chem. Soc.*, 65, 1273, 1943.
62. **Steinhausen, T. B., Dungan, C. E., Furst, J. B., Plati, J. T., Smith, S. W., Darling, A. P., Wolcott, E. C., Warren, S. L., and Strain, W. H.**, Iodinated organic compounds as contrast media for radiographic diagnoses. III. Experimental and clinical myelography with ethyl iodophenyl-undecylate (Pantopaque), *Radiology*, 43, 230, 1944.
63. **Ramsey, G. H., French, J. D., and Strain, W. H.**, Iodinated organic compounds as contrast media for radiographic diagnoses. IV. Pantopaque myelography, *Radiology*, 43, 236, 1944.
64. **Camp, J. D.**, Contrast myelography past and present, *Radiology*, 54, 477, 1950.
65. **Peacher, W. G. and Robertson, R. C. L.**, Pantopaque myelography, results, comparison of contrast media and spinal fluid reaction, *J. Neurosurg.*, 2, 220, 1945.
66. **Bering, E. A.**, Notes on retention of Pantopaque in subarachnoid space, *Am. J. Surg.*, 80, 455, 1950.
67. **Erikson, T. C. and van Baaren, H. J.**, Late meningeal reaction to ethyliodophenylundecylate used in myelography; report of case that terminated fatally, *JAMA*, 153, 636, 1953.
68. **McLaurin, R. L.**, Myelomalacia and multiple caviations of spinal cord secondary to adhesive arachnoiditis, *Arch. Pathol.*, 57, 138, 1954.
69. **Arabuckle, R. K.**, Pantopaque myelography: correlation of roentgenologic and neurologic findings, *Radiology*, 45, 356, 1945.
70. **Hobbs, M. L.**, Meningitis due to pseudomonas aeruginosa followig myelography with Pantopaque, *W. V. Med. J.*, 53, 180, 1957.
71. **Tarlov, J. M.**, Pantopaque meningitis disclosed at operation, *JAMA*, 129, 1014, 1945.
72. **Wyatt, G. M. and Spurling, R. G.**, Pantopaque: notes on absorption following myelography, *Surgery*, 16, 561, 1944.
73. **Kieffer, S. A., Peterson, H. O., Gold, L. H. A., and Binet, E. F.**, Evaluation of dilute Pantopaque for large-volume myelography, *Radiology*, 96, 69, 1970.
74. **Rubin, M. and diChiro, G.**, Chelates as possible contrast media, *Ann. N.Y. Acad. Sci.*, 78, 764, 1959.
75. **diChiro, G. and Fisher, R. L.**, Contrast radiography of the spinal cord, *Arch. Neurol. Chicago*, 11, 125, 1964.
76. **Fisher, R. L.**, An experimental evaluation of Pantopaque and other recently developed myelographic contrast media, *Radiology*, 85, 537, 1965.

77. **Borrelli, F. J. and Maglione, A. A.,** The importance of myelography in spinal pathology, *Am. J. Roentgenol.,* 76, 273, 1956.
78. **Belenger, J., Simons, M., Jeanmart, L., and Danis, A.,** Evolution de la myelographie, *J. Belge Radiol.,* 54, 347, 1971.
79. **White, A. G.,** Prolonged evaluation of serum protein-bound iodine following myelography with Myodil, *Br. J. Radiol.,* 45, 21, 1972.

Chapter 3B

II. WATER-SOLUBLE CONTRAST MEDIA

The development of water-soluble contrast media began with the introduction of sodium mono-iodo-methane sulfate by Arnell and Lindström in 1931.[1] The utilization of water-soluble contrast media for myelography came as a result of unfavorable experiences and reports about the noxious effects of iodized oils. The study published by Odin and Runström in 1928, spurred an intensive research aimed at substituting the iodized oil with a contrast medium that would be nonirritant, water-soluble, miscible with the spinal fluid, and which would have considerable opacity and capability to be absorbed and eliminated without deleterious aftereffects. Excellent studies concerning the application of such contrast agents published first by Arnell and Lindström in 1931, Arnell in 1944, Lindblom in 1946, and the classical work of Arnell published in 1948, promoted the usage of water-soluble contrast media for myelography.[1-4] After a rather enthusiastic reception of mono-iodo-methane sulfate, it became nonetheless evident that its application was limited because it caused a severe irritating effect on the meninges and nerve roots, and could be used only in combination with lumbar anesthesia for the exploration of the lower lumbar and sacral areas. These serious limitations of the first water-soluble contrast medium were the reason why it was not generally accepted. It was evident that the introduction of water-soluble contrast media did not solve the problem of contrast agents for myelography that could be used without noxious side effects.[27,33-35]

Since the introduction of the first water-soluble agent for myelography, almost to the present time, a division of opinion has persisted, namely, in some institutions radiopaque insoluble contrast media were used exclusively, and in others, water-soluble contrast agents were utilized for the exploration of the lumbar and sacral areas. In essence, the available radiopaque contrast media fell short of optimal requirements and the choice of the radiopaque contrast medium was more a matter of opinion and developed myelographic techniques than the question of qualitative superiority of the medium itself. The advantages and disadvantages of different soluble and nonsoluble contrast media have become the theme of a profuse literature that has not resolved this issue.[7,11,13,30] The first absorbable, hydrosoluble, hyperbaric contrast medium sodium mono-iodo-methane sulfate (Abrodil®, Methiodal®, Kontrast U®, Skiodan®, Myelotrast®, etc.) had the capability to outline on radiographs, in a clear and detailed fashion, the nerve roots and the lumbar subarachnoid space and thus became the contrast agent of choice for radiculography. The frequent side effects connected with this type of myelography were attributed to the injection of the contrast medium and to the spinal anesthesia.[17] The injection of mono-iodo-methane sulfonic acid into the lumbar subarachnoid following spinal anesthesia could provoke pain that would appear excruciating, and headaches that occurred almost invariably and would last sometimes up to 3 to 7 days. Moreover, convulsions and unconsciousness, increased root pain for one or more days, diffused pain in the lower extremities, abdominal and back pain of shorter or longer duration, vomiting, nausea, contractures, severe collapse, and even death were reported.[34,35] The more common side effects such as headache and some degree of pain had less clinical significance than the occasional saddle block anesthesia, incontinence, and other complications described by different authors and attributed to lumbar anesthesia.[30,34-36] Funkquist conducted an experimental study with Kontrast U® 20% applying 1.5% Xylocaine® for lumbar anesthesia. The dogs used for this experimental work showed signs of neurological deficit such as paresis of legs. The recording of the blood pressure indicated that a moderate fall in blood pressure after the injection of the contrast medium did not give rise to any serious functional disturbances or histopathologic changes. A marked fall in blood pressure, however, after the injection of the contrast medium with otherwise identical experimental conditions, was the cause of a severe spinal cord damage in most animals. The morphologic changes in the spinal cord consisted of a focal edema localized to white matter, and in some, edematous foci, a central area of necrosis was observed.[27] Changes of the position of the animals after the injection of the contrast medium may have aggravated the fall in blood pressure, especially if the injection was combined with lumbar anesthesia (Xylocaine®).

The exchange of the fluid between the capillaries and the extracellular spaces in the CNS is highly sensitive to the changes in the osmotic pressure of the blood. The question whether the contrast medium exerts its injurious effect mainly by osmosis or by more specific toxic properties was studied by different authors.[26-28,31] Concerning the functional and morphologic signs of spinal cord lesions, injection of saline was found to produce damage of the same type and degree of severity as the injection of the contrast medium that had an identical osmotic pressure and was injected under similar conditions. As far as the effect on the blood-spinal cord barrier was concerned, the increase in capillary permeability to trypan blue was only slightly reduced after the injection of saline 5.1% than after the injection of Kontrast U® 20%. Such comparative studies of the subarachnoid injection of the saline solution and the contrast medium, respectively, suggest that the noxious effect of the medium depends upon osmotic factors. Some studies indicated that the changes in the blood-spinal cord barrier after the subarachnoid injection of water-soluble contrast media showed an abrupt increase in capillary permeability when the concentration of the medium was raised from 15 to 20%.[31-33]

Neurotoxicity of the first water-soluble contrast agents for myelography derived, in essence, from iodobenzoic acids and their osmotic activity and solubility of the lipids.[42] The later synthesis of polymeric derivatives of the anionic component of the contrast medium resulted in a reduction of this osmotic activity and consequently in toxicity. The disclosure and understanding through many experimental works of this mechanism prompted the search for a new water-soluble contrast medium that could be used for the exploration of the lumbar subarachnoid space with fewer hazards.

The research in the area of water-soluble contrast media for myelography produced the sodium-free contrast agent meglumine iothalamate (Conray®), introduced by Campbell in 1962. The introduction of meglumine iothalamate was received with great interest, especially after Campbell's second publication in 1964.[7] Meglumine iothalamate could be used for the exploration of the lumbar subarachnoid space without anesthesia. The introduction of this type of water-soluble contrast medium was preceded by extensive laboratory work by different authors with diatrizoate (Urografin®), acetrizoate (Jodozoat®, Trijotyl®, Urokon®) and iodopyracet (Diodon®, Per-Abrodil®). Later in 1966, Hilal described the dimer of meglumine iothalamate known as iocarmate meglumine (Dimer X®). The work done by Gonsette in 1968 and 1971, Baumegarden and co-workers in 1968, Davies and co-workers in 1968, Legre and co-workers in 1968, and Grainger and co-workers in 1971, opened a new era in the development of more suitable water-soluble contrast media, and a controversial attitude concerning the contrast agents for myelography, that had remained unchanged for more than 30 years, became less marked. Many radiologists converted to water-soluble myelography for it produced excellent radiographic visualization of the lumbo-sacral nerves and their root sleeves.[6,8-11,16]

Meglucamine iothalamate and meglucamine iocarmate had an appreciable neurotoxicity, and with few exceptions, most investigators limited examinations to the conus medullaris and the lumbosacral nerve roots. The three types of water-soluble contrast media used: methiodal sodium (Abrodil®, Kontrast U®, etc.), meglumine iothalamate (Conray®, etc.) and meglumine iocarmate (Dimer X®, Bis-Conray®, Dimeray®, etc.) had not gained general acceptance because of their irritative effects upon the nervous structures.[20,22,25,26]

Mycoclonic spasms were recorded after the injection of meglucamine iothalamate and meglucamine iocarmate as well as headaches, vomiting, neck stiffness, increased regional pain in the lumbar region, hypotension, and paresthesias. Anatomo-pathologic studies carried out with these two water soluble contrast media (Contrix 28® and Dimer X®) by Gonsette in 1971, and other investigators, indicated that vasodilation with edema and a rather severe inflammatory reaction of the spinal cord occurred under the influence of Conray® and less of Dimer X®. Gonsette, in his biological study, advocated that the dilution of Contrix 28® was preferable for the usage in myelography to the original concentration.[16] This study, as well as others, confirmed, however, that these two contrast media were less noxious and caused less damage to the meninges and spinal cord than the previously used methiodal (Abrodil®).[12] Both of these contrast media had a tendency to produce a localized arachnoiditis, and some investigators utilized steroid compounds mixed with the contrast medium to reduce the inflammatory reactions.[27] Arachnoiditis noticed on myelograms in the lumbar area was manifested by root shortening of different degrees and/or rounding off of root sheaths, or by more extensive involvement of the meninges in the cranial direction. The percentage of pathologic arachnoid changes after the injection of Contrix® showed no correlation with the recorded levels of spinal fluid protein. Some investigators recommended in order to avoid arachnoiditis, the removal of these contrast media after the examination if a high protein content had shown. However, this procedure was of little value. Ahlgren mixed 5 mℓ of Dimer X®, 2 mℓ of spinal fluid and 2 mℓ of steroids for lumbar myelography.[26] Apparently, the incident of late arachnoid changes increases after myelography with Contrix®, Conray®, and Dimer X® in that order. Although Dimer X® had less incidence of headaches and immediate reactions than Conray®, and less than 1% of subsequent clonic spasms, its later effect on the meninges was discouraging. Adding steroids to Dimer X® did not give the anticipated advantage of preventing the occurrence of arachnoid adhesions.[5,12,14,15,29]

The studies done by Speck et al. concerning the passage of meglumine iocarmate (Dimer X®), ioserinate (Myelografin® and Metrizamide®) into the blood after lumbar myelography produced interesting results.[25] The side effects recorded during and after the lumbar myelography with these water-soluble contrast media appeared to be related to the technique of the procedure (lumbar puncture, low cerebrospinal pressure syndrome) and, to some extent, to the direct effect the contrast medium had on the nervous system. A direct neurotoxic action of the contrast medium is to be expected only for as long as the CSF actually contains the contrast agent. Therefore, a number of investigators had paid special attention to the distribution, transport, and resorption of the contrast agent using conventional radiography, computed tomography, isotope scanning, and measuring the concentrations of the medium in the body fluids.[20-22]

According to the observations of Cécile et al. in 1974, Dimer X® is more quickly absorbed from the CSF and causes fewer side effects if the patient remains in bed lying down after the examination.[22] The effect of the posture of the patient and the velocity of the passage of the contrast medium from the CSF into the blood has been a matter of discussion. Namely, if the patient is placed in an approximately horizontal position immediately after the injection of the contrast medium into the lumbar area, the transport of the contrast agent apparently starts earlier, hence its blood level also rises sooner. According to our own observations concerning this matter, as well as those of other investigators, it may be assumed that the distribution of the contrast media in the subarachnoid space and mixing with the CSF is a prerequisite for the agent's transfer into the blood. Such distribution has actually been demonstrated by isotope scanning and by computer tomography after lumbar injection. The transport of contrast agents from the CSF into the circulatory system may occur through an active mechanism which was demonstrated in the choroid plexus of the ventricles and on the convexity of the brain.[24] The CSF produced in the choroid plexus was believed to flow out through a pressure operated valve mechanism in the cranial and spinal arachnoid villi. The arachnoid villi have three valve-like openings about 2 to 12 μm in diameter. Mixed with CSF itself, any dissolved substance may get into the venous blood. Essentially, the velocity of transport from the subarachnoid space would depend on the time necessary for the CSF secretion, the CSF dynamics, and the miscibility of the contrast medium. The outflow and circulation of the CSF could be influenced by the change in the position of the patient from the vertical to the horizontal. The half-life of the transfer of the water-soluble contrast medium from the CSF into the blood is approximately 3.9 to 2.4 hr. Thus the speed of elimination is mostly accomplished in about 24 hr. The velocity of transport, however, varies considerably from one patient to another. It appears that the water-soluble contrast media flow passively when mixed with the CSF through the arachnoid villi into the venous blood.[23-25]

Such analyses of the effect of the above mentioned contrast media as well as those related to the usage of mono-iodo-methane sulfate (Abrodil®, Kontrast U® 20%, etc.) were discouraging and caused considerable hesitation concerning the application of water-soluble contrast agents.[26-28,36,37]

A possible solution to some problems related to the water-soluble contrast media used for myelography came in 1969 with Almén's proposal of the synthesis of a nonelectrolytic water-soluble contrast medium.[32] One year later, Oftedal described a new contrast medium with lower toxic effects when injected intrathecally in experimental animals.[36] This nonelectrolytic, water-soluble medium called Metrizamide® (Amipaque®) was based on a new principle for the synthesis of water-soluble contrast agents, and was introduced by Almén in an attempt to use the nonionic compounds in order to decrease the osmolarity of the previously applied water-soluble contrast media, since hypertonicity was probably the main cause of some adverse and noxious effects of these contrast agents. Based upon Almén's proposal, a series of nonionic compounds was synthetized and one of these substances, namely Metrizamide®, was found to be less noxious. It was therefore chosen for further investigation. More than 3 years of intensive laboratory studies with a view on pharmacology, toxicology, and physiology preceded its use in humans. On the basis of these studies, Metrizamide® was found to have a rather low toxicity and a lesser irritative effect on the CNS and meninges when introduced into the subarachnoid spaces of experimental animals.[18,19,21,38-42]

REFERENCES

1. **Arnell, S. and Lindström, F.**, Myelography with Skiodan (Abrodil), *Acta Radiol. Diagn.*, 12, 287, 1931.
2. **Arnell, S.**, Weitere erfahrungen über myelographie mit Abrodil, *Acta Radiol. Diag.*, 25, 408, 1944.
3. **Lindblom, K.**, Lumbar myelography by Abrodil, *Acta Radiol. Diagn.*, 27, 1, 1946.
4. **Arnell, S.**, Myelography with water-soluble contrast, with special regard to the normal Roentgen picture, *Acta Radiol. Suppl.*, 75, 1, 1948.

5. **Occleshaw, J. V. and Holyland, J. N.**, Comparative study of the effects of Conray 280 and Dimer X in lumbar myelography, *Br. J. Radiol.*, 44, 946, 1971.

6. **Baumegarten, J., Braun, J. P., Rust, F., Wipf-Scheibel, M., Kummert, J., and Kiesel, R.**, Amélioration de la technique de l'examen radiculographique par utilisation d'un nouveau produit de contrast, *Neuro-Chir.*, 8, 909, 1968.

7. **Campbell, R. L., Campbell, J. A., Heimburger, R. F., Kalsbech, J. E., and Mealey, J.**, Ventriculography and myelography with absorbable radio-opaque medium, *Radiology*, 82, 286, 1964.

8. **Davies, F. M., Llewellyn, R. C., and Kirgis, H. D.**, Water-soluble contrast myelography using meglumine iothalamate (Conray) with methylprednisone acetate (Depro-Medrol), *Radiology*, 90, 705, 1968.

9. **Gonsette, R. and Andre-Balisaux, G.**, New technique for lumbo-sacral myelography using a water-soluble contrast media without root anesthesia, *Ann. Radiol.*, 11, 141, 1968.

10. **Legre, J., Salamon, G., Altan, D., Lavielle, J., Guidicelli, G., and Dufor, M.** Nouvelle technique de myéloradiculographie avec contraste iodehydrosoluble résorbable sans rachianésthesie, *Presse Med.*, 76, 1707, 1968.

11. **Grainger, R. G., Gumpert, J., Sharpe, D. M., and Carson, J.**, Water-soluble lumbar radiculography, a clinical trial of Dimer X — a new contrast medium, *Clin. Radiol.*, 22, 57, 1971.

12. **Praestholm, J. and Lester, J.**, Water soluble contrast myelography with meglucamine iothalamate (Conray), *Br. J. Radiol.*, 43, 303, 1970.

13. **Gonsette, R.**, Water-soluble contrast media in neuroradiology, *Clin. Radiol.*, 22, 44, 1971.

14. **Schmiedel, E.**, Die lumbosacrale Myelographie mit Einem neuentwickelten kontrastmittel, *Der Radiol. Berl.*, 12, 478, 1970.

15. **Hammer, B. and Scherrer, H.**, Choice of contrast medium in lumbrosacral myelography, *Neuroradiology*, 4, 114, 1972.

16. **Gonsette, R.**, Utilisations nouvelles des produits de contraste hydrosolubles en neuroradiologie, *J. Belg. Radiol.*, 54, 385, 1971.

17. **Bidstrup, P.**, A case of chronic adhesive arachnoiditis after lumbar myelography with methiodal-sodium, *Neuroradiology*, 3, 157, 1972.

18. **Evill, C. A. and Benness, G. T.**, Urographic excretion studies with metrizamide and "Dimer" a high dose comparison in dogs, *Invest. Radiol.*, 12, 169, 1977.

19. **DiChiro, G. and Schellinger, D.**, Computed tomography of spinal cord after lumbar intrathecal introduction of metrizamide (computer assisted myelography), *Radiology*, 120, 101, 1976.

20. **Braband, H., Lessman, H. D., and Wenker, H.**, Experimentelle Untersuchungen uber die Elimination und Neurotoxisität Eines neuen Wasserlöslichen Kontrastmittels zur lumbosakralen Myelographie, *Radiologe*, 12, 66, 1972.

21. **Goman, K.**, Absorption of metrizauide from cerebrospinal fluid to blood: pharmacokinetics in humans, *J. Pharm. Sci.*, 64, 405, 1975.

22. **Cécile, J. P., Regnier, G., Guadquière, A., Doffiny, L., and Cuvelier, A.**, Postural protection against complications in radiculography with Dimer X, *Neuroradiology*, 7, 167, 1974.

23. **Cserr, H. F.**, Physiology of the choroid plexus, *Physiol. Rev.*, 51, 273, 1971.

24. **Schneider, M.**, *Physiologie des Menschen*, Springer-Verlag, New York, 1966.

25. **Speck, U., Schmidt, R., Volkhardt, V., and Vogelsang, H.**, The effect of position of patient on the passage of metrizamide (Amipaque), meglumine iocarmate (Dimer X) and ioserinate (Myelografin) into the blood after lumbar myelography, *Neuroradiology*, 14, 251, 1978.

26. **Ahlgren, P.**, Long term side effects after myelography with water soluble contrast media: Conturex, Conray Meglumin 282 and Dimer X, *Neuroradiology*, 6, 206, 1973.

27. **Funkquist, B. and Obel, N.**, Effect on the spinal cord of subarachnoid injection of water-soluble contrast medium, *Acta Radiol. Diagn.*, 56, 449, 1961.

28. **Pag, K. M. and Wheeler, D. O.**, Water-soluble lumbar radiculography, *Radiography*, 452, 194, 1972.

29. **Haidenthaler, W. and Kollar, A. F.**, Erfahrungen mit Conray — Myelographien, *Radiol. Clin. Biol.*, 41, 65, 1972.

30. **Lange, J. and Odegaard, H.**, Abrodil myelography in herniated disk in lumbar region, *Am. J. Roentgenol.*, 57, 186, 1951.

31. **Hilal, S. K.**, Hemodynamic changes associated with the intraarterial injection of contrast media. New toxicity tests and a new experimental contrast medium, *Radiology*, 86, 615, 1966.

32. **Almén, T.**, Contrast agent design. Some aspects on the synthesis of water soluble contrast agents of low osmolality, *J. Theor. Biol.*, 24, 216, 1969.

33. **Halaburt, H. and Lester, J.**, Leptomeningeal changes following lumbar myelography with water-soluble contrast media (Meglumine iothalamate and methiodal sodium), *Neuroradiology*, 5, 70, 1973.

34. **Johansen, A. H.**, Todesfall nach einer myelographie mit Per-Abrodil *Nord. Med.*, 17, 163, 1943.

35. **Karlen, A.**, Todesfall an Fettknochenmarkembolie und Uramie nach "intraduraler" Per-Abrodil myelographie, *Acta Chir. Scand.*, 87, 497, 1942.

36. **Oftedal, S. T.,** Meningeal reactions to water-soluble contrast media in cats, *Acta Radiol. Suppl.,* 335, 153, 1973.
37. **Praestholm, J.,** Experimental evaluation of water soluble contrast media for myelography, *Neuroradiology,* 13, 25, 1977.
38. **Skalpe, T. O. and Amundsen, P.,** Lumbar radiculography with Metrizamide, *Radiology,* 115, 91, 1975.
39. Introduction — Metrizamide, *Acta Radiol Diagn. Suppl.,* 335, 1973.
40. **Nickel, A. R. and Salem, J. J.,** Clinical experience in North America with metrazamide. Evaluation of 1850 subarachnoid examinations, *Acta Radiol. Diagn. Suppl.,* 335, 409, 1977.
41. **Barry, J. F., Harwood-Nash, D. C., Fitz, C. R., Sharon, B. E., and Boldt, D. W.,** Metrizamide in pediatric myelography, *Radiology,* 124, 409, 1977.
42. **Hilal, S. K., Danth, G. W., Hess, K. H., and Gilman, S.,** Development and evaluation of a new water-soluble iodinated myelographic contrast medium with markedly reduced convulsive effects, *Radiology,* 126, 417, 1978.

Chapter 3C

III. CHEMICAL PROPERTIES OF OPAQUE CONTRAST MEDIA

Chemical properties of most commonly used absorbable and not absorbable contrast media will be discussed here briefly. Less commonly utilized contrast agents, or those the use of which had been discontinued, have been already mentioned in the introduction of this chapter.

Pantopaque®, presently used, according to its manufacturer, represents a mixture of isomers of ethyl iodophenylundeconoate. The compound is colorless or a pale yellow liquid containing 30.5% of organically bound iodine. The specific gravity of ethyl iodophenylundecanoate is about 1.26 at 20°C. Pantopaque® has the tendency to change color in sunlight, but it can be stored without deterioration for a long period of time. Its usage is specifically recommended for myelography. The suggested amount of Pantopaque® to be injected into the subarachnoid space is 3 to 12 cc. In some instances, however, a large quantity is required in order to outline the subarachnoid space.

Metrizamide® (Amipaque®, made by Nyegaard in Norway) was synthesized as a water-soluble, nonionic tri-iodinated medium for lumbar, thoracic, and cervical myelography. Metrizamide®, as well as Pantopaque®, has also been used for ventriculography. It has been applied experimentally as a contrast agent for epidurography, and it appears to be well tolerated in this procedure due to its low toxicity.[1] The conventional ionizing water-soluble contrast media, all of which are salts, have a higher osmolarity than Metrizamide®, which is not a salt. The synthesis of Metrizamide® represents a new approach in the development of contrast media based on the assumption that different toxic effects of previously used water-soluble contrast agents are related to their hyperosmolarity. As Metrazamide® does not have the tendency to dissociate in an aqueous solution, its solutions have a considerably lower osmolarity, about one third less than other water-soluble contrast agents.[2,9,10]

Metrazamide® is a compound derived from the metrizoic acid and glucosamine with molecular weight of 789, and a content of iodine of 48.25%. The organically bound iodine gives the necessary opacity to this contrast medium. The experimental work carried out with Metrizamide® suggests that at 20 to 30°C, a solution of 80 g/100 ml can be obtained, which makes it highly soluble in water. The solution of Metrizamide® in comparison to ionic compounds of the same iodine content have a slightly higher viscosity. With vapor pressure instruments, the osmolarity of blood and Metrazamide® solution had been determined, and the results showed that the Metrizamide® solution containing 170 mg iodine per milliliter was basically isotonic with human blood and with CSF. The density of Metrazamide® is somewhat higher than the one of the normal CSF.[2-11]

The contrast media containing iodine used for myelography are generally sensitive to light, including Metrizamide®. Iodine, if exposed to light, is inclined to split off in its inorganic form. In order to achieve such an effect, the exposure to the direct sunlight is the most effective, although the diffuse daylight may have the same impact on iodine. Therefore, it is advised that Metrizamide's dry substance be stored in such a way that it is protected from daylight, or even from the light of electric lamps.[2]

The exposure of iodine containing contrast agents to the primary irradiation has to be avoided. The secondary irradiation that occurs in a radiologic diagnostic setting is apparently of less importance, and does not considerably affect the iodine compounds.[4]

Metrizamide® is absorbed rather fast from the CSF, and the peak of the serum concentrations were determined experimentally to be about 1 to 2 hr after suboccipital injection in cats.[3] In the body fluids of different experimental animals, the distribution of labeled Metrizamide® was approximately similar to that of labeled diatrizoate and other angiographic contrast agents.[17] The biologic half-life of Metrizamide® is 0.6 to 2.2 days in the tissues of the experimental animals, except in the thyroid gland where it lasts to about 5 days.[5-7] According to a number of experimental studies as well as clinical observations, Metrizamide® is excreted mainly in the urine, and to a lesser extent in the bile.[7-13] The laboratory studies indicated that Metrazamide® caused less aggregation and less paradoxical hypertonic hemolysis than some other contrast media.[15-18] Salversen in 1973 demonstrated experimentally that Metrazamide® inhibited less the enzyme activity than ionic contrast media.[15] Metrizamide® apparently does not affect gluconeogenesis, but glycolysis is reduced by about 25%.[17,19]

Following the lumbar intrathecal injection of Metrazamide®, it was possible to detect its presence in blood 15 min later. The peak concentration of Metrazamide® in the serum occurs approximately 2 hr after the subarachnoid injection in humans, and approximately 50% of the injected dose of Metrazamide® disappears from the CSF in about 1 hr.[5]

The possibility of following the absorption and flow of Metrazamide® after the lumbar injection by means of computed tomography was demonstrated by Greitz and Hindmarsh in 1974 and 1975.[11,20] These studies suggest that Metrizamide® could be eliminated in man by diffusion through the meningeal membranes or by transport with the CSF through its pathways. It seems that the diffusion is predominant with contrast media that have a low molecular weight (methiodal sodium), and that the CSF transport is more common with contrast media of higher molecular weight (meglumine iocarmate, Metrizamide®).

Metrizamide® (Amipaque®) is provided by the manufacturer as a sterile, white lyophilized powder. The vials contain 3.75 g of Metrazamide® (1.81 g organically bound iodine) and 1.2 mg edetate calcium disodium, or 6.75 g of Metrazamide® (3.26 g organically bound iodine) and 2.16 mg edetate calcium disodium. Each 20 mℓ vial of sterile aqueous dilutent contains 0.05 mg/mℓ sodium bicarbonate in the water with pH adjusted with carbon dioxide. When Metrazamide® is reconstituted to the lowest recommended concentration of 170 mg I/mℓ its gravity counts 1.814 at 37°C; it is hyperbaric to CSF; it is iostonic with CSF; and has a pH of about 7.4.

Following the subarachnoid instillation, Metrizamide® will provide an adequate radiopacity on radiographs, usable for diagnostic purposes, for approxiamtely 1 hr. Later, radiopacity becomes hazy and the Metrizamide® is not detectable 24 hr following the subarachnoid injection. An upward diffusion of Metrizamide® takes place though the CSF following the subarachnoid instillation, regardless of the position of the patient.[11]

The utilization of Metrizamide® should be reconsidered in patients with known hypersensitivity to iodine, in patients with epilepsy, severe cardiovascular diseases, chronic alcoholism, and multiple sclerosis. If a history of allergy is established, premedication with antihistamines may be considered. It is advisable to continue the anticonvulsant therapy in patients who are under such treatment, and should a seizure occur in patients who are not undergoing epileptic treatment, intravenous diazepam is recommended. If a larger amount of Metrizamide® enters inadvertently into the intracranial subarachnoid space, a prophylactic anticonvulsant treatment with barbituates or diazepam should be considered.[14] Any drugs, such as neuroleptics and phenothiazine derivatives which lower the seizure threshold, should be avoided, and the administration of such medications discontinued at least 48 hr before myelography, and 12 hr after the procedure.[21] Patients with hepatorenal insufficiency should not have a Metrizamide® myelography unless the benefit of this diagnostic procedure outweighs the additional risk. Repeated myelography with Metrizamide® should be delayed for about 7 days or more.

Concerning some pharmacologic and biologic effects of Metrizamide®, it should be mentioned that epileptic activity was demonstrated in experimental animals awakening from anesthesia.[21] The seizures were attributed to the interaction between Metrizamide® and chlorpromazine. Also, the occurrence of meningeal adhesions was reported. Apparently, the addition of blood to Metrizamide® did not alter the severity of arachnoid adhesions.[22,23]

REFERENCES

1. **Kido, D. K., Schoene, W., Baker, R. A., and Rumbaugh, C. L.,** Metrizamide epidurography in dogs, *Radiology*, 128, 119, 1978.
2. **Holtermann, H.,** Metrizamide, Introduction, *Acta Radiol. Diagn.*, Suppl. 335, 1, 1973.
3. **Golman, K. and Dahl, S. G.,** Absorption of labelled metrizamide, diatriozate, inulin and water from cerebrospinal fluid to blood, *Acta Radiol. Diagn.*, Suppl. 335, 276, 1973.
4. **Shussler, R.,** Der Jodidgehalt jodirter wasserlöslicher Röntgenkontrastmittel und seine veränderung durch Röntgenstahlen, *Fortsch. Röntgenstr.*, 97, 649, 1962.
5. **Golman, K.,** Absorption of metrazamide from cerebrospinal fluid to blood: pharmacokinetics in humans, *J. Pharm. Sci.*, 64, 405, 1975.
6. **Frey, K.,** Thin-layer chromatography of 125T-labelled metrazamide in urine from laboratory animals, *Acta Radiol. Diagn.*, Suppl. 335, 268, 1973.
7. **Golman, K. and Scient, C.,** Metrazamide in experimental urography, *Invest. Radiol.*, 11, 187, 1976.
8. **Anumdsen, P. and Skalpe, L. O.,** Cervical myelography with water-soluble contrast medium (Metrizamide). A preliminary clinical report with special reference to technical aspects, *Neuroradiology*, 8, 209, 1975.
9. **Gonsette, R. E.,** Metrizamide as contrast medium for myelography and ventriculography. Preliminary clinical experiences, *Acta Radiol. Diagn.*, Suppl. 335, 346, 1973.
10. **Hindmarsh, T.,** Myelography with the non-ionic water-soluble contrast medium metrizamide, *Acta Radiol. Diagn.*, 16, 417, 1975.
11. **Hindmarsh, T.,** Elimination of water-soluble contrast media from the subarachnoid space, *Acta Radiol. Diagn.*, Suppl. 346, 45, 1975.
12. **Hindmarsh, T.,** Methiodal sodium and metrizamide in lumbar myelography, *Acta Radiol. Diagn.*, Suppl. 335, 366, 1973.
13. **Valk, J.,** Myelography with metrizamide (Amipaque), *Medicaumndi*, 21, 164, 1976.
14. **Gonsette, R. E.,** Biological tolerance of the central nervous system to metrizamide, *Acta Radiol. Diagn.*, Suppl. 335, 25, 1973.
15. **Salversen, S. and Frey, K.,** Protein binding of metrizamide and the effect on various enzymes, *Acta Radiol. Diagn.*, Suppl. 335, 247, 1973.
16. **Almén, T.,** Angiography with metrizamide. Animal experiments and preliminary clinical experiences, *Acta Radiol. Diagn.*, Suppl. 335, 419, 1977.
17. **Almén, T., Boijsen, E., and Lindell, S. E.,** Metrizamide in angiography. I. Femoral angiography, *Acta Radiol. Diagn.*, 18, 33, 1977.
18. **Almén, T.,** Influence of pH of metrazamide on hypotension following intraaortic injection, *Acta Radiol. Diagn.*, Suppl. 335, 203, 1973.
19. **Munthe-Kaas, A. C. and Seglen, P. O.,** The use of metrizamide as a gradient medium for isopycnic separation of rat liver cells, *FEBS Lett.*, 43, 252, 1974.
20. **Greitz, T. and Hindmarsh, T.,** Computer assisted tomography of intracranial CSF circulation using a water-soluble contrast medium, *Acta Radiol. Diagn.*, 15, 497, 1974.
21. **Gonsette, R. E. and Brucher, J. M.,** Potentiation of Amipaque. Epileptogenic activity by neuroleptics, *Neuroradiology*, 14, 27, 1977.

22. **Haughton, V. M., Ho, K. C., Larson, S. J., Unger, G. F., and Correa-Paz, F.,** Experimental production of arachnoiditis with water-soluble myelographic media, *Radiology,* 123, 681, 1977.
23. **Haughton, V. M., Ho, K. C., Larson, S. J., and Correa-Paz, F.,** Arachnoiditis following myelography with metrazamide in monkeys. Effect of blood in the cerebrospinal fluid, *Acta Radiol. Diagn.,* Suppl. 355, 373, 1977.

Chapter 4

MYELOGRAPHIC TECHNIQUE WITH INSOLUBLE CONTRAST MEDIA*

Myelography technique with radiopaque, insoluble contrast media could be divided into several steps: selection of radiologic equipment, positioning of the patient, puncture of the subarachnoid space and injection of the contrast medium, radiographic-fluoroscopic exploration, removal of the contrast medium, and the patient care after myelography. Each step is of an equal importance for a successful performance of myelography. To consider myelography as a simple procedure that can be carried out under unfavorable conditions might lead to technical and diagnostic errors, and to clinical complications.

Prior to myelography, it is advisable to become familiar with the patient's clinical signs and the course of his disease. Some clinical details can influence the site of the puncture, technique of injection, decision about the type and removal of the contrast medium, and the radiographic technique.

The choice of radiologic equipment for myelography is of consequence because it should provide the possibility of fluoroscopy and controlled radiography, lateral and cranio-caudal movements of the table top, tilting of the table so that the patient can be easily positioned in the Trendelenburg and upright postures. The presently used equipment is generally supplied with the image amplification and television, as well as with a spot film device for radiography under fluoroscopic control. The possibility to perform cineradiography in selected cases is an asset since it permits a precise reconstruction of the fluoroscopic picture and it acts as a "frozen memory".[1] It is rather preferable to have a special radiographic room for myelography which should, if possible, serve only for this purpose. However, as this is not often the case, at least no barium enemas, genito-urinary radiologic procedures, or fistulography should be conducted in this setting. The sterility in the room designated for myelography should abide by the same rules as those applied to the operating rooms. In this way, the possibility of contamination of the meninges will be considerably reduced.

A close collaboration with the attending neurologist, neurosurgeon, or orthopedic surgeon before and after myelography is advantageous for mutual understanding of radiologic findings, and for a fast communication in case of undesirable side effects that can be traced to the myelography or the disease. This type of teamwork within neurosciences is generally accepted and it helps the tasks of neuroradiology.

In the Fifties, we used chiefly the "small quantity technique" injecting 3 to 6 cc of the oily insoluble contrast medium (Myodil®) into the lumbar subarachnoid space. After the injection the needle would be withdrawn and the patient positioned for fluoroscopy and radiography. The contrast medium was not removed. This technique, still used by many investigators, shortens the myelographic procedure and is much better tolerated by the patient. However, its disadvantage is not negligible since the contrast medium remains dwelling within the subarachnoid space after the examination for an indefinite period of time.

Since the early Sixties up to the present time, we have been applying the puncture of the lumbar subarachnoid space with the patient in the prone position, and the subsequent removal of the contrast medium has been carried out if indicated. The utilization of the specially designed sponges, different in shape and size, will facilitate the

---

* References for this chapter appear at the end of Chapter 5.

positioning of the patient. Before the patient is placed in the prone position, a sponge, triangular in shape, is placed on the table so that it may compress the patient's anterior abdominal wall and arch his back in the lumbar area. An adjustable footrest attached to the radiographic table provides the necessary support to the patient's feet. A shoulder support covered with soft material or a canvas sling will prevent the movement of the patient's body in the cranial direction in the course of the examination of the thoracic and cervical areas. Additional sponges or soft pads are inserted under the patient's shoulder, knee, or at other appropriate areas, depending upon the radiographic technique. Proper positioning will permit the performance of the examination with a minimal displacement of the patient's body. If the patient feels as comfortable as the conditions allow, he will be more relaxed, his muscles in the region of the back less contracted and thus the puncture simplified. The displacement of the patient with the needle in the lumbar subarachnoid space is avoided for it can cause a movement of the needle itself, and the widening of the puncture site in the meninges could result in the leakage of the CSF or eventually of the contrast medium. Furthermore, the patient's own moving can cause bending of the needle, displacement of its position, perforation of the anterior wall of the subarachnoid space, penetration of the needle into the epidural space, laceration of epidural or other veins, puncture of the nerve roots, and it may also be the cause of difficulties during the removal of the contrast medium.

It is of considerable importance to explain to the technologists the whole procedure step by step, and to keep at least one technologist permanently attached to the myelographic room. The examiner should be familiar with the chemical and pharmacologic properties of the contrast medium before myelography begins, and the selection of the needle for the puncture of the subarachnoid space should be carefully determined. A variety of needles of different widths and lengths are available for lumbar and suboccipital punctures. Since 1968 we have been using the Cuatico® set with a thin wall 18-gauge spinal needle and a blunt end aspiration cannula with multiple side holes.[2,3] Using this needle, the unpleasant pain that the patient could experience in the course of the withdrawal of the contrast medium after myelography was eliminated.

In order to reduce the skeletal muscle spasm in the lumbar region ensuing from a reflex spasm connected to local pathology (disk), we had good experience with an intramuscular injection of 5 to 10 mg of diazepam (Valium®). A local anesthesia (Novocaine® 1%, Xylocaine® 1%) of the skin and deep muscles of the region selected for puncture would provide an adequate analgesia that would further relax the muscles and facilitate the puncture. It is postulated that the cellular reaction occurring within the CSF could be allergic in nature and the administration of antihistaminic agents (Benadryl® 50 mg, or similar compounds) could eventually prevent or decrease some changes in the CSF seen following the injection of the contrast media into the subarachnoid space. Equally, the injection of steroids apparently decreases the number of the cells in the CSF.

Careful consideration is given to the selection of the interspace for the entry of the needle. In general, one avoids the space most likely to harbor the pathologic process since the needle itself may produce a filling defect that could be the cause of diagnostic errors. Probably the best choice for the entry is at the L_2 to L_3 interspace, that is, above the imaginary line between the iliac crests usually indicating the level of L_4. It is advisable to determine the exact level of the interspace under fluoroscopy and to mark on the skin the site of puncture. Ordinarily, we would use a 3- to 3.5-in. long needle, 18 gauge, or a 4-in. long needle if the patient is obese. In children, the same type of needle only shorter (21 or 20 gauge) would be used. We apply a midline puncture, and only in some instances, for example in case of extensive ossified postoperative scars, an oblique approach would be considered. A precise midline placement of the needle advanced ventrally, and for a few degrees cranially into the subarachnoid space so that the tip almost touches the ventral theca, will help avoid subdural injection of the contrast agent and facilitate its recovery. It is safest to perform the puncture under the control of fluoroscopy. If the needle is not in the midline, it can bypass the dura and come in contact with the nerve roots, which can be a painful experience for the patient. In this case, the needle should be withdrawan, the position of the patient checked, and a second attempt of puncture made under fluoroscopic control. If the needle is in a good position, the sharp stylet is removed and a free flow of spinal fluid will appear. If the flow is not abundant or intermittent, the needle should be gently readjusted with the rotation to the right and left or reinserted for another milimeter. If a good flow of the spinal fluid is obtained, the free end of the needle is connected to a 50-cm long sterile plastic tube (different types of venous extension tubes are available) provided with a valve at the free end (3-way plastic stopcock). Subsequently, an opening pressure can be recorded as well as the effect of the jugular compression and the release test (Queckenstedt). We would carry out these tests in exceptional situations to determine an eventual obstruction of the spinal canal if the fluid was yellow or its flow inadequate. About 5 cc of the spinal fluid is allowed to collect in the thin-walled test tubes for laboratory determination of the cells, protein, and eventually other analyses. Following this, the valve on the tube is closed. We prefer to have the valve attached to the tube and not to the needle because the metallic valve will make the free end of the needle much heavier and therefore influence the change of the needle's position. If the needle is well installed in the subarachnoid space, any further maneuvers with the needle should be avoided (Figure 1).

A 20-cc syringe is filled with 12 cc of the contrast medium, warmed to body temperature, and attached to the free end of the plastic tube. The valve is opened and with a gentle pressure under the control of fluoroscopy, about 0.5 to 1 cc of the contrast medium is injected. If the needle is in a good position, the injected contrast medium will move promptly and freely up and down in the subarachnoid space. The movements of the contrast medium will be accentuated if the patient is asked to cough softly, or if the table is tilted.

If the position of the needle appears correct after the test injection of the contrast medium, the table is raised gently with jerky movements for about 45°, and the contrast medium slowly injected under fluoroscopic control. The amount of the contrast medium depends upon the adopted myelographic technique, age of the patient, width of the subarachnoid space, pathologic process, and site of puncture. We would inject 12 cc of the contrast medium if the spinal canal was free. However, if the spinal fluid had a yellow color and manometric readings, and Queckenstedt test indicated an obstruction, we would inject about 2 to 4 cc of the contrast medium that would not be removed after the examination. Occasionally, a larger amount of the contrast medium may be necessary and it can be added in the course of the examination. Exceptionally, we would apply the so-called full column technique with 30 or more cc of the contrast medium. A larger amount of the contrast medium can obscure a small lesion and cause some difficulties in the interpretation of the radiographs. Important to mention, however, is the fact that the injected contrast medium will accumulate on the ventral surface of the subarachnoid space due to the gravity, and if the circumference of the spinal canal needs to be visualized, the patient ought to be placed in an accentuated oblique or eventually supine position. The supine position requires the removal of the needle and a second puncture in order to recover the contrast material. The amount of the contrast agent has to be sufficient to carry out a good study according to the adopted myelographic technique (Figure 2).

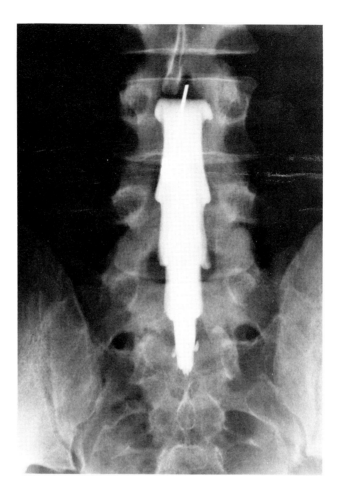

FIGURE 1. In the anteroposterior position on this lumbar myelogram, the subarachnoid space in the lumbosacral area is shown filled
with Pantopaque®. The nerve roots are outlined and the shape of the
caudal end of the arachnoid sac clearly marked. Note the midline
placement of the needle directed slightly cranially.

The injection of the contrast medium should be done slowly so that it flows in a
steady stream to avoid globulation of the oily substance. If the injection is successfully
performed, the plastic tube is disconnected and the stylet replaced in the needle. The
needle is covered with a sterile towel securely fixed with an adhesive tape to the patient's body (Figure 3).

If difficulties are encountered in the course of the puncture or injection of the contrast medium, and the attempts to remove the obstacle are not successful, persistence
should be avoided. It is preferable to terminate the examination and after a period of
approximately 10 to 14 days repeat the procedure.

The spot film device should be fixed by an adjustable lock so that it cannot come in
contact with the needle or the sterile towel. The exploration of the subarachnoid space
is carried out by means of fluoroscopy and radiography which are inseparable and
thus combined can provide the best diagnostic results. The movement of the contrast
medium in the subarachnoid space is scrutinized under fluoroscopy. The spot films
are taken at different intervals. Standard radiographs in lateral, oblique, and other

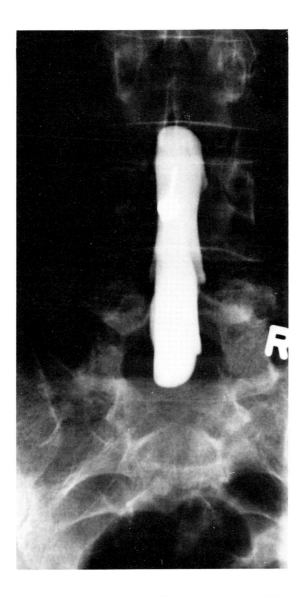

FIGURE 2. Slow lumbar instillation of opaque insoluble contrast medium following the test injection. The table is raised for about 40° and the contrast flows freely. The caudal end of the arachnoid sac is not yet outlined. The nerve roots are visible encircled by the meningeal sleeves. Observe the position of the needle.

positions are performed following fluoroscopy, spot film radiography, and/or cine-myelography (Figure 4).

The evaluation of the *lumbo-sacral area* is done with the patient in an almost upright position of the table. Spot films under fluoroscopic control are carried out with the patient in the anteroposterior, right and left oblique projections. Additional oblique projections under different angles might be necessary and a lateral projection is added with the patient in the erect position. For a lateral film, only a horizontal beam should be utilized. By tilting the table gradually from the upright to the horizontal and Trendelenburg positions, the opaque column of the contrast medium will be moved to the

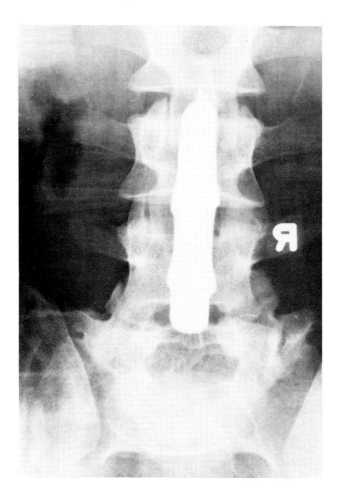

FIGURE 3. The injection of Pantopaque® was done slowly to
avoid globulation. By tilting the table higher up, the lower portion of
the subarachnoid space was filled with the contrast medium. The radiopaque contrast concentrated in one area in the larger quantity covers the nerve roots.

lower thoracic area. Each interspace should be demonstrated in anteroposterior,
oblique, and lateral projections. In addition to these standard views, different optional
projections can be applied. For example, if the patient is in hyperextension in the erect
position, the ventrodorsal diameter of the subarachnoid space could be reduced by the
bulge of the ligamentum flavum and annulus. A radiograph in the posteroanterior
projection with the caudal angulation of the tube for about 20° proved to be sufficient
for the study from the L_5 to S_1 interspace. For the detection of minor defects of the
nerve root sleeves, right and left lateral decubitus radiographs, obtained with the horizontal beam and grid cassette, are helpful. It should be emphasized that radiographs
of the lower thoracic area should be obtained at least up to T_9 because the demonstration of this region is an integral part of lumbar myelography (Figure 5).

   For the visualization of the pathologic process in the *thoracic area,* a larger amount
of the contrast medium is suggested by some authors.[1,4] Others, on the other hand,
prefer to carry out the examination with smaller quantities of an opaque medium of
12 cc or less. If the table is carefully and gradually tilted cranially, the contrast medium

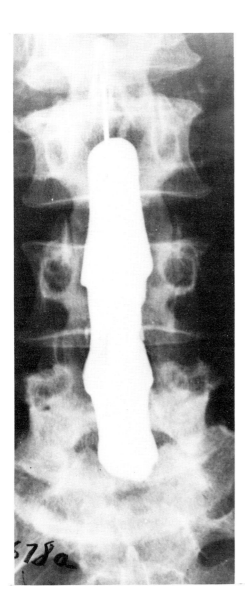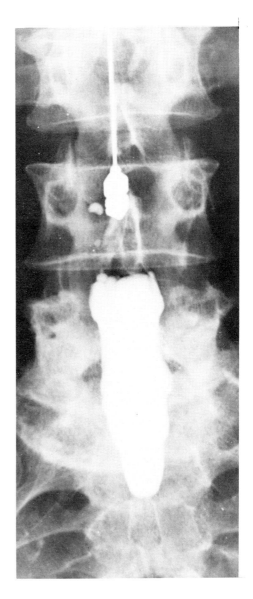

A   B

FIGURE 4. (A). Pantopaque® myelogram in anteroposterior projection, with the table tilted upwards for 35°, does not delineate the caudal end of the arachnoid sac. This incomplete filling may cause an erroneous impression that the distal part of the sac is short or obstructed. (B). If the table is tilted higher head-up, the contrast medium will descend and the caudal end of the arachnoid sac will assume its shape and length. (C). If the filling of the caudal end of the arachnoid sac is incomplete, it may appear narrowed or compressed. These technical errors are easily corrected by bringing the patient in an upright posture.

will flow in a steady stream, especially in the oblique position of the patient. Right and left accentuated oblique and/or lateral projections are important for the examination of the thoracic area. In these positions, in our experience, lesions can be detected with greater precision. The patient's head must be elevated and extended. It is not necessary to tilt the table more than about 25 to 30° in the cranial direction to obtain a good uninterrupted flow of the contrast medium to the thoracic subarachnoid

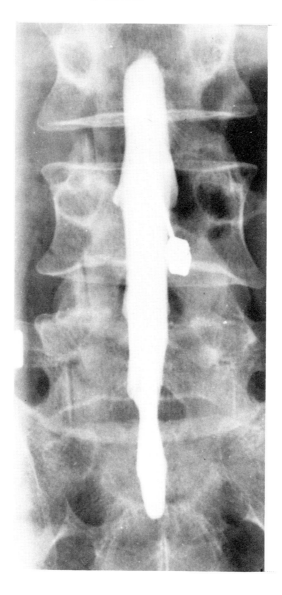

FIGURE 4C.

space. A careful fluoroscopic control of the movements of the contrast medium through the thoracic subarachnoid space is imperative. Spot radiographs should be used at appropriate intervals and in different positions if a lesion is suspected. The application of cinemyelography is especially helpful for the investigation of the thoracic area. If the contrast medium begins to break into droplets, which occurs often in the thoracic region, especially around T_5, it is possible, occasionally, to bring the column together by compressing the jugular veins. The contrast medium will form an elongated compact radiopaque column, and the examination of the thoracic area will be possible. In other instances, it might be preferable to bring the droplets of the contrast material into the cervical area and let the opaque column descend from the cervical into the thoracic region by tilting the table caudad.[9] After fluoroscopy and spot radiography, standard radiographs of the thoracic spine are obtained in the posteroanterior, cross-table lateral, and both oblique projections. Infrequently, the patient has

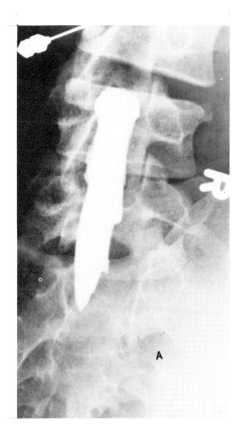

A

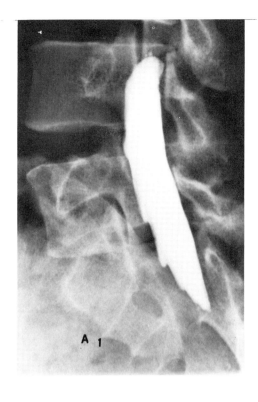

B

A

FIGURE 5. (A, B, C). Lumbosacral myelogram with the patient in an almost upright position, in right and left oblique projections. In oblique positions the nerve roots and meningeal sleeves are accessible to scrutiny and can be evaluated more precisely. The pictures demonstrate the appearance of the lumbosacral subarachnoid space and different angles of the patient's rotation. (D, E). More accentuated oblique positions delineate the relationship between the subarachnoid space and the spinal canal. The prominent nerve roots are seen in Figure E. (F). Appearance of the subarachnoid sac in the lumbosacral region in oblique views filled with a smaller quantity of oily contrast medium (6 cc).

to be turned into the supine position after the removal of the needle so that some pathologic changes (A-V malformation or small neurinoma) attached to the posterior surface of the spinal cord or in the posterior compartment of the subarachnoid space can be demonstrated. The exploration of the thoracic space includes the lower cervical and upper lumbar areas as well (Figure 6).

The myelography of the *cervical region* comprises the visualization of the foramen magnum, cisterna cerebellomedullaris (magna), cisterna pontis up to the interpeduncular cistern. Further passage of the contrast medium can be impeded by the membrane of Liliequist. The contrast medium should not penetrate into the middle or anterior cranial fossae for it is practically impossible to remove it from these areas. The cervical myelogram should demonstrate clearly the margins of the foramen magnum because some pathologic processes in this region can produce clinical signs that might be indicative of a lesion in the upper cervical area. In view of this, a cervical myelogram should be considered incomplete if the base of the posterior cranial fossa is not visualized (Figures 7, 8).

Before the exploration of the cervical region, the support of the patient's shoulders

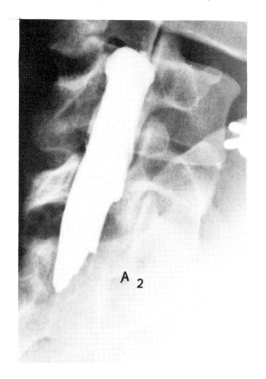

FIGURE 5C

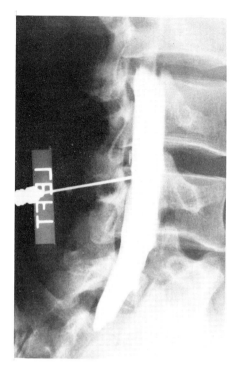

FIGURE 5D

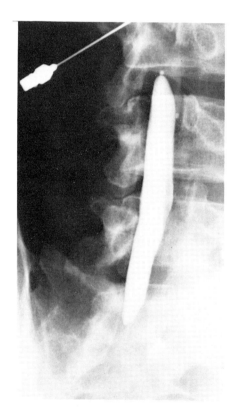

FIGURE 5E

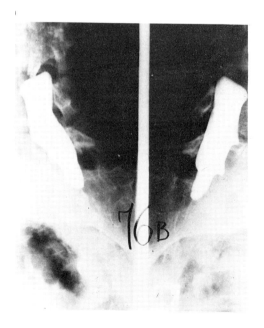

FIGURE 5F

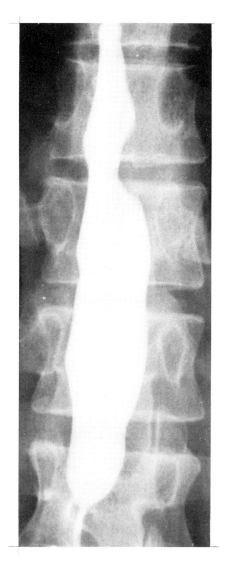

A

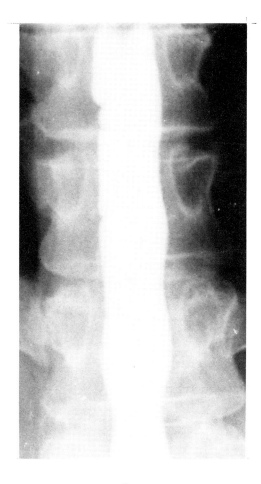

B

FIGURE 6. (A). The column of the oily contrast medium in the thoracic area tends to break into larger or smaller drops and streaks in the prone position. (B). If the table is gradually tilted head-down under control of fluoroscopy for about 25 to 30°, an uninterrupted flow of the contrast will be obtained. The anterior spinal artery is often seen if the contrast medium is evenly distributed in a thinner layer. (C). The contours of the spinal cord and nerve roots will be more apparent if the contrast is spread over a longer thoracic segment.

should be fixed. The patient's head is positioned in hyperextension. If the patient is slightly turned into an oblique position, the flow of the contrast medium will be facilitated. With the further gentle tilting of the table into a head-down position of about 30°, the cervical subarachnoid space will be gradually filled with the complete amount of the injected contrast medium. The foramen magnum and the base of the posterior fossa are explored, and spot radiographs obtained. Occasionally, slight rotation of the patient's head to the right and left is required to fill in the cisterns with the contrast medium. Following this, the table is brought into an almost horizontal position, and

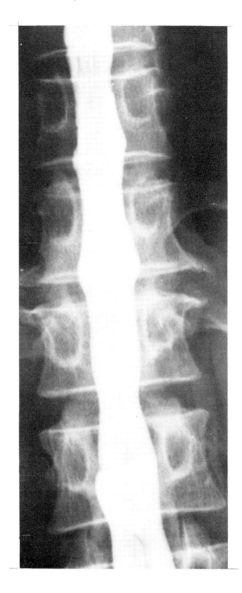

FIGURE 6C

the exploration of the cervical canal is done under fluoroscopic control in oblique and prone projections during this part of the examination. The neck of the patient is in a flexed, neutral, and extended position. The examination of the lower part of the cervical subarachnoid space should always cover the upper thoracic area. Spot films and cineradiography are most useful for the evaluation of the cervical region. The routine radiographic views for the cervical area consist of posteroanterior and two or three cross-table lateral projections. Under different circumstances, it is also necessary to bring the patient's head into a more flexed or extended position, which is generally done by the examiner with his lead-gloved hands. In the process of such examinations, additional radiographic positions might be required (Figures 9, 10).

For a good demonstration of C_6 or C_7 and the first thoracic vertebrae, the cross-table lateral films can be obtained with the patient's shoulder dropped as low as possible. Usually, the examiner gently pulls the hands of the patient in the caudal direc-

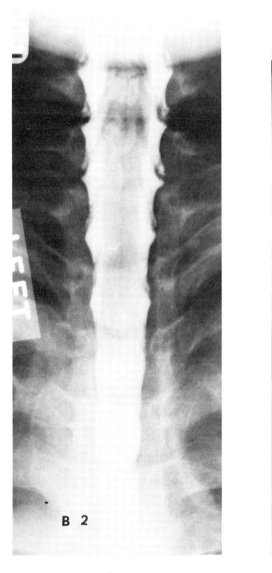

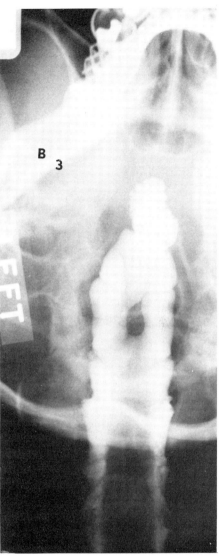

A   B

FIGURE 7. (A). Myelogram in the prone position of the patient shows a gradual uninterrupted flow of Pantopaqe® through the upper thoracic and lower cervical regions. With gentle tilting of the table into a head-down position for approximately 30° under fluoroscopic control, the thoracocervical junction and the cervical subarachnoid space are gradually filled with the full amount of the injected contrast medium. (B). The patient's head in the prone position is in hyperextension and the cervical subarachnoid space filled with Pantopaque.®. The oval radiolucency of the dens is well demonstrated. The anterior spinal artery is seen in both figures and the spinal cord with exiting nerves is visible too. Small spondylotic spurs are visualized in Figure A.

tion. The swimmer's position is particularly important. Sometimes, it may be difficult to advance the column of the contrast medium into the cervical region if spondylosis and narrowing of the spinal canal are present. Turning the head into an oblique position, the obstacle can generally be bypassed. Some difficulties may also occur owing to the break up of the contrast medium into smaller droplets in the cervical area. Further obstacles to the flow of the contrast medium can be the unwillingly performed

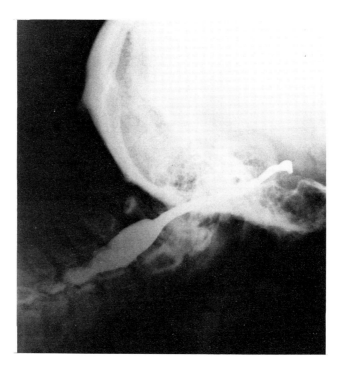

FIGURE 8.   Myelogram of the upper cervical area and the base of
the skull outlines the cisterna pontis. The column of the contrast medium completely filled the subarachnoid space to the end of the dor-
sum sellae, but it did not penetrate into the cisterna chiasmatica, interpeduncularis, or Sylvii.

Valsalva maneuver, by the patient himself or an increased pooling of venous blood in
the epidural plexus if the patient is in an accentuated Trendelenburg position. Consequently, a cervical obstruction noticed in the Trendelenburg position cannot be considered as certainty if not confirmed with radiographs in horizontal, oblique, and cross-
table lateral projections. Regarding the flow of the contrast medium in the region of
the posterior fossa, the penetration of the oily substance above the tentorial notch into
the middle fossa will not occur if the apex of the notch is higher than the upper end
of the contrast column. The posterior margin of the foramen magnum should be visualized, and, if necessary, the needle removed and the patient placed in the supine
position when this cannot be achieved in oblique projections (Figure 8).

Standard radiographies of a specific area or of the whole spine precede each myelography. These radiographs should be carefully analyzed because some congenital or
acquired anomalies can be readily detected and may influence the course of myelography. Equally important is the evaluation of the radiographs obtained during the myelographic procedure. It is advisable to check a set of radiographs of one area of the
spine before the contrast medium is moved to the next. The decision about additional
projections should be made at the moment of the first inspection of radiographs because the fluoroscopic impression will be fresh in memory at the time, and the area in
question can be reexamined if necessary. A good collaboration with the patient should
be established before myelography and maintained during its course. In this way, the
patient is confident and feels more comfortable about the whole examination. In the
course of the procedure, it is good to talk to the patient and let him know what is
going on at a certain point in time.

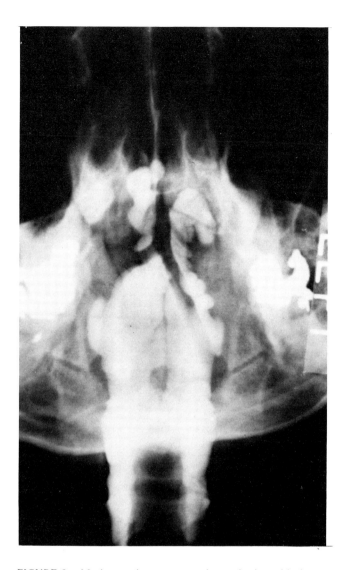

FIGURE 9. Myelogram in anteroposterior projection with the patient in the prone position. The head is hyperextended and the contrast medium fills the area of cervicocranial junction. The vertebral arteries and the origin of the basilar and anterior spinal arteries are clearly outlined. The contrast flows on both sides of the basilar artery into the cisterna pontis. The incorrect marking of the patient's side can happen, as illustrated in this figure.

If a pathologic process is detected, its location should be precisely marked on the radiographs by fixing lead numbers on the patient's skin laterally at the level of the lesion. Generally, we would mark one vertebral body above and one below the process involved. We use numbers because they indicate accurately the level of the vertebral body, which is particularly important in the thoracic area. Often, it is necessary to mark the lower and upper pole of the lesion by lead markings, especially if the patient is considered for surgical treatment. The central part of the lesion involved can be marked on the skin of the patient by a superficial scratch with a sterile needle. In this way, a possible misunderstanding about the exact level of the lesion can be avoided, and the surgeon feels more confident about the interpretation of different indicators

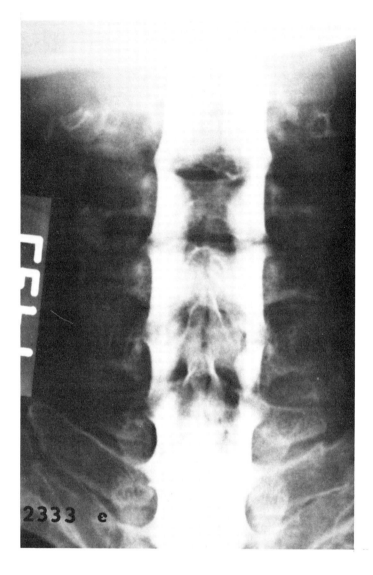

A

FIGURE 10.   (A). Following the exploration of the base of the skull, the table is brought into an almost horizontal position and the examination of the cervical canal is done under fluoroscopic control. In the patient's prone posture the spinal cord and nerves are clearly seen because the contrast medium is spread evenly in the subarachnoid gutters. The intervertebral spaces may be more prominent, particularly if discreet spondylotic ridges are present. (B, C). The examination of the cervical region should be conducted also in the right and left oblique positions. (D). By tilting the table gently higher up under fluoroscopic control, the contrast medium is brought again into the distal cervical and proximal dorsal region. This area is explored once more in anteroposterior oblique and "swimmer's" views (see normal myelogram).

on the radiographs. If surgery is considered after myelography, it is advisable to discuss with the surgeon involved the results of this diagnostic procedure. The patient should be comfortable in the course of the examination to avoid straining that can considerably diminish the width of the canal in some persons. It is possible to estimate approximately the width of the canal from the flow of the CSF. If the tip of the needle is in a good position and the flow of the spinal fluid intermittent, one should assume that the canal is narrow.

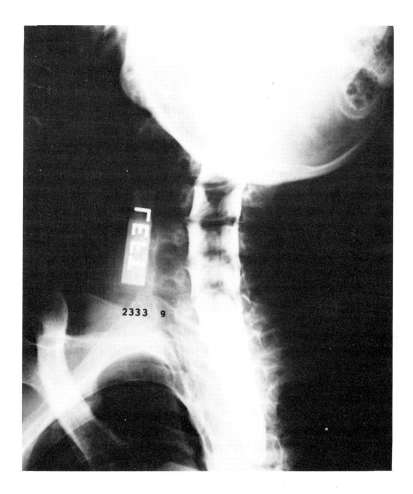

FIGURE 10B

In elderly patients with severe spondylosis, or in some other skeletal, congenital, or acquired changes, the lumbar puncture could be rather difficult. In this case, a *trans-sacral puncture* of the arachnoid sac may be considered. Several techniques had been described for the trans-sacral puncture of the arachnoid sac. More recently, Haverling in 1972 described a good approach to this area.[5] Although we have used the sacral approach in some instances, we believe that in most cases it is possible to carry out a lumbar puncture with an appropriate technique. Often, we carried out the instillation of the contrast medium into the subarachnoid space using the *cisternal puncture*. The injection of the contrast medium into the cisterna magna is performed in case the lumbar puncture cannot be achieved; to outline the upper pole of a lesion obstructing the subarachnoid space; to demonstrate multiple lesions in the sinal canal; and if the patient could not be placed in the prone position due to his disease. In quadriplegics, for example, the suboccipital approach can be technically the easiest and least disturbing to the patient. In order to perform efficiently the suboccipital myelography, a precise positioning of the patient is important. The patient is placed in a correct left lateral decubitus with his head in an anterior flexion so that the chin almost reaches the chest. The occipital area and the upper part of the neck should be shaved and the procedure carried out as any other myelography under strictly sterile conditions. The head is placed on a soft pad or sponge so that it is exactly parallel with the surface of the table. The position of the head is checked on fluoroscopy. Following the cleaning

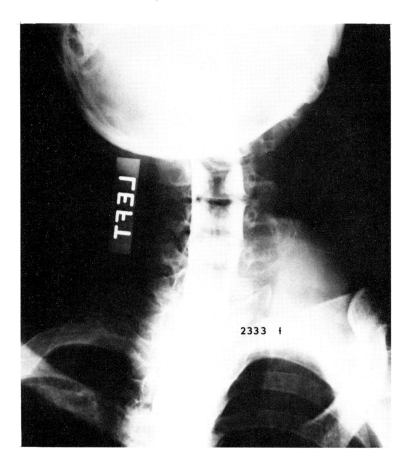

FIGURE 10C

of the skin and draping of the area with sterile gloves above the drapes, both mastoid processes are felt and the midpoint of an imaginary line connecting the two processes is found. The point is punctured with a needle for the cutaneous injection and checked under fluoroscopy. Through the same needle, 1% Xylocaine® or some other local anesthetic is injected to provide good analgesia of the skin and neck muscles. Different needles can be used for the suboccipital puncture. We found that a shorter Cuatico® type of needle was convenient for this procedure, although we had good experience with some other types as well. It is important that the needle is not heavy, especially not the free end that is attached to the plastic tube. It is helpful to perforate the skin at the site of puncture with a short 18- or 17-gauge needle, for this will facilitate the passage of the needle for the subarachnoid puncture. After the opening of the skin at the junction of the line extending from the external occipital protuberance to the midpoint of the imaginary line that connects the two tips of mastoid processes, the needle for the cisternal puncture is inserted precisely parallel to the surface of the table. The needle is directed gently forward as well as cranially under fluoroscopic control between the occipital bone and the C_1 vertebral body. An elastic resistance is sensed as the tip of the needle touches the dura. The perforation of the dura is distinctly felt and the needle is advanced a few milimeters forward. The stylet is removed from the needle, and if the needle is in a good position, an abundant, free flow of CSF will occur. At this point, the plastic tube is attached to the needle and the table carefully raised up for about 20°. Approximately 0.5 to 1.0 cc of the contrast medium is slowly

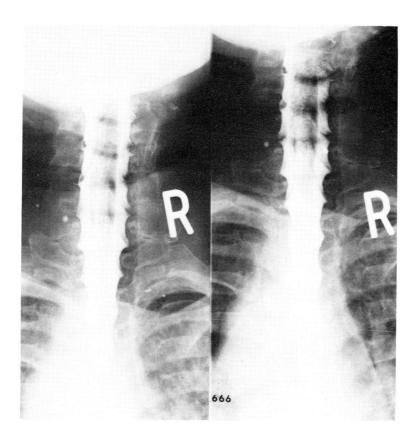

FIGURE 10D

injected under the control of fluoroscopy. The contrast agent will flow freely in the cisterna magna and descend into the upper part of the cervical subarachnoid space. If any resistance is noticed, further injection should be stopped immediately and the flow of the spinal fluid checked. Sometimes, it may be necessary to carefully readjust the position of the needle. The amount of the contrast medium injected into the cisterna magna and the subarachnoid space is usually less than the amount injected into the lumbar area. In most instances, about 6 to 8 cc will suffice to outline the subarachnoid space in the upper cervical or thoracic areas.

A *lateral cervical puncture* can be used instead of the suboccipital. We had equally good experience with this approach using mostly the technique described by Shapiro, Mullan, and Kelly and Alexander.[4,6,7] According to their technique, the patient is in the supine position with the head elevated for approximately 10°. Under fluoroscopic control, the site of puncture between C_1 and C_2 is marked precisely on the skin. After the local anesthesia is achieved (Xylocaine® 1%, Novocaine® 1%), under sterile conditions, the needle is inserted and its advancement followed on the television screen. In the supine position, the spinal cord is displaced dorsally and the anterior compartment of the subarachnoid space becomes somewhat wider. As the needle reaches the dura, there is a response of an elastic resistance. The needle is advanced carefully forward into the anterior subarachnoid compartment and the stylet removed. If the needle is in a good position, a free flow of the CSF will appear. The position of the needle can be checked on radiographs. If the flow of the spinal fluid is free, the plastic tube is attached to the needle and about 0.5 cc of the contrast medium is instilled under fluoroscopic control. If the contrast medium moves freely in the subarachnoid space in the course of this test injection, the main instillation can follow. The total amount of the contrast medium varies, and depends upon the technique and pathologic process. About 6 cc is generally sufficient. In the course of the main injection of the contrast medium, the table is tilted slowly upwards in the caudad direction. The lateral approach may not, however, be feasible if edema or tumor of the spinal cord are present, or obvious pathologic changes of the bony structures. In the latter case, the cisternal puncture might be a better choice. The contrast medium injected by means of cisternal or lateral cervical puncture is not removed. In both cases, standard radiography of the appropriate area is carried out following the fluoroscopic exploration and spot film radiography. If difficulties are encountered with cisternal or lateral cervical punctures, it is not opportune to insist and repeat the punctures because it is possible to damage a smaller blood vessel or the nervous tissue. It is more appropriate to interrupt the procedure and consider a second attempt approximately 1 week later.

A *transcoronal puncture* of ventricles with the injection of about 2 cc of the contrast medium in infants, with subsequent maneuvers to direct its flow into the third and fourth ventricle and the spinal subarachnoid space, under fluoroscopic control, was described by Salmon.[8] This technique is used in case of different pathologic processes when the lumbar or suboccipital punctures may not be feasible.

A number of additional myelographic techniques have been described in the literature. The choice of the technique depends largely upon the experience gained with one of them, as well as on the specific situation faced at the time of the exploration of the spinal subarachnoid space. If the lumbar puncture is not possible in case of expansive epidural or subdural lesions, diffuse arachnoiditis, low CSF pressure due to multiple punctures, epidural, subdural or subarachnoid hemorrhage, etc. a different route for the injection of the contrast medium should be contemplated.

The removal of the contrast medium after the lumbar instillation is performed under fluoroscopic control. The blunt stylet with side holes, attached to the plastic tube, is gently inserted through the needle into the subarachnoid space. The table is tilted in the cranial and caudad direction until the contrast medium is accumulated in one column around the needle's tip. At times, before the aspiration begins, approximately 1 to 2 cc of air from the syringe can be injected to detach the nerve roots from the needle and the stylet. The aspiration of the contrast medium with the Cuatico® type of needle is relatively simple. It should be done slowly, carefully rotating the piston of the syringe and gradually moving it upwards. In the course of the aspiration, the position of the table is adjusted with slow movements in such ways that the contrast medium remains around the needle's tip. If the patient complains of pain, the aspiration should stop, the needle carefully readjusted with rotating movements, and eventually additional air injected. After a successful removal of the contrast medium, a radiograph of the lumbar region is obtained to confirm the absence of the contrast medium in the subarachnoid space. Many techniques have been described for the evacuation of the contrast medium related, especially, to the utilization of heavy iodized oils such as Lipiodol®.[5] For example, good results have been attained with technique of syphonage introduced by Epstein.[1] If the contrast medium cannot be removed due to an intensive pain, a second puncture, at a lower interspace, can be performed and the contrast medium collected usually from the L_5 to S_1 region. A suction of a larger amount of the spinal fluid should be avoided by slightly advancing the needle in the ventral direction and collecting the contrast medium around the bevel by tilting the table in the appropriate direction. Sometimes, the column of the contrast medium may break up and it might be difficult to collect smaller and larger drops. In this situation, the table should be tilted upwards so that the contrast material accumulates in the caudad end of the subarachnoid space. When this is accomplished, the table is slowly tilted in the craniad direction and the contrast brought again around the needle in one solid column. Difficulties in removing the contrast medium will occur if the needle is not in the central position. In this situation, the patient should be placed in an oblique posture and supported with rubber sponges so that the collecting of the contrast material in the subarachnoid gutter, closer to the bevel of the needle, may take place. If the difficulties in removing the contrast medium persist and the patient complains of a severe pain, it is probably best to terminate these attempts, to remove the needle, and after a week or more perform a second puncture at the L_5 to S_1 interspace.

If the myelograms are not conclusive, the injected contrast medium can be left in the subarachnoid space for several days, and the examination can be repeated without injecting the contrast agent for the second time. Following the reexamination, the lumbar puncture at L_5 to S_1 is performed and the contrast medium removed. In case of complete obstruction, the contrast medium is left in the subarachnoid space and the patient can be reexamined. On this second examination, the contrast medium occasionally can outline, in a more satisfactory way, the lower pole of the lesion, and eventually bypass the obstruction in a narrow stream, completely or partially. In this case, it is important to tilt the cephalad end of the table as far as possible under the control of fluoroscopy, and in addition to the spot radiographs, exposures with a horizaontal beam and grid cassette are obtained in the lateral and frontal positions. If the contrast medium is injected into the cisterna magna, a reexamination is helpful because the obstruction can be visualized more clearly if the patient remains for 1 or more days with his back elevated. Beside spot radiographs, the cross-table lateral projection is required in case of this reevaluation.

When an obstruction is present, it is not uncommon that the contrast medium stops at a certain distance from the lower pole of the lesion and thus fails to outline faithfully its surface. The cause of obstruction will be actually higher than the block demonstrated by the column of the contrast agent. By using a maximum tilt of the table under fluoroscopic control and spot film radiography followed by frontal and lateral radiographs, this error can be avoided most of the time. If the contrast medium is not removed, it is advantageous to reexamine the patient before surgery to be certain that the level of the lesion is correctly outlined. A high level of protein in the spinal fluid (1000 mg or more per 100 mℓ) contributes to the slow flow of the contrast medium and to its complete stop below the level of the lesion.

Prior to myelography, no puncture of the subarachnoid space for the purpose of collecting the spinal fluid for laboratory and monometric readings should be done, because a leakage of the CSF can occur in the subdural and epidural spaces. The leakage can be the cause of errors at the time of the lumbar puncture for myelography, since the flow of the spinal fluid from the needle is not indicative of the needle's correct position in the subarachnoid space. The injected contrast medium under these circumstances can be distributed in the epidural, subdural, and subarachnoid spaces. Myelography should not be carried out sooner than 10 to 15 days after the lumbar puncture was performed, except if it is absolutely imperative for clinical or other reasons.

Upon the removal of the contrast medium, the patient should remain flat in his bed for about 24 hr to avoid the postlumbar puncture headache. It is advantageous to explain to the patient why he should be in the horizontal position and warn him about the headache, which can be controlled with analgesics. It may be useful to recommend a fluid diet for the patient since a larger amount of fluids tends to decrease the incident and severity of the postlumbar puncture headache. The orders for the patient's care should be noted in the chart, and it is customary to follow the course of a patient's symptoms and signs for about 1 or 2 days. We would require the laboratory to send a copy of the findings in the CSF so that the laboratory sheet could be attached to the radiologic procedure sheet.

Chapter 5

MYELOGRAPHIC TECHNIQUE WITH RADIOPAQUE WATER-SOLUBLE CONTRAST MEDIA

Myelography technique with radiopaque, absorbable water-soluble contrast media differs from the techniques applied for myelography with insoluble contrast agents. Several myelographic techniques were described using as a contrast medium sodium *mono-iodo-methane sulfate* (Kontrast U®, Abrodil®, etc.). We have used this compound in combination with lumbar anesthesia in over 1200 lumbar myelographies in the following way. The lumbar puncture was performed with the patient in a sitting position at the level of L_4 to L_5. About 5 to 6 cc of the spinal fluid were collected for laboratory examination. After this, the patient was placed on his left side on top of the table tilted for approximately 45° in the caudad direction, and the lumbar anesthesia was performed. Following the lumbar anesthesia, the patient was not moved in order to avoid the possibility of an abrupt collapse. The effect of the lumbar anesthesia was checked, and under fluoroscopic control, 1 to 2 cc of the contrast medium were injected. If no reaction occurred, and the contrast medium appeared to be instilled into the subarachnoid space, the main injection followed. Approximately 10 cc of the contrast medium were injected and the needle withdrawn. Under fluoroscopy, with the table elevated for about 30 to 25°, spot films were exposed in the lateral, oblique, and prone positions. Following this part of the examination, standard anteroposterior, oblique and cross-table lateral radiographs were obtained. The examination was carried out rather fast because of the rapid elimination of the contrast medium (Figure 1).

The introduction of *meglumine iothalamate* (Conray®) and *meglumine iocarmate* (Dimer X®, Dimeray®, Bic-Conray®) simplified the myelographic procedure since there was no need for anesthesia. Both contrast media were used mainly for the exploration of the lumbar region. Upon the instillation of these contrast media under fluoroscopic control, the needle was withdrawn and the examination performed in a similar way as described above. A detailed description of myelographic techniques utilizing the above mentioned water-soluble contrast agents will be omitted in this text because they have become obsolete since the introduction of *Metrizamide®*.

With the application of Metrizamide®, the preparation of the patient consists of an intramuscular injection of 5 to 10 mg of diazepam (Valium®), although some examiners do not give any premedication.[35,36] A local anesthesia is performed (Xylocaine® 1%, Novocaine® 1%) preceding the lumbar puncture because the muscle contractions of the patient's back are thereby reduced and the puncture facilitated. Some examiners do not use local anesthesia. Spinal anesthesia with the use of Metrizamide® is contraindicated. A corticosteroid and/or antihistamine premedication is suggested in patients who have a history of hypersensitivity to iodine or different allergic dispositions. It should be noted that all phenothiazine derivatives as well as some other compounds discussed earlier ought to be avoided in conjunction with Metrizamide® myelography.[10,15,36]

Preparation of the Metrizamide® solution should be done under sterile conditions prior to the myelographic procedure. A 10- or 20-cc syringe is filled with the exact volume of the solvent as indicated on the attached chart. One should add 8.9 mℓ of the solvent to the vial containing 3.75 g of Metrizamide® to obtain a 170 mg I/mℓ solution, and 16.1 mℓ of the solvent to the vial containing 6.75 g of Metrizamide® to achieve the 170 mg I/mℓ solution.[35,36] The air must not penetrate into the vial before

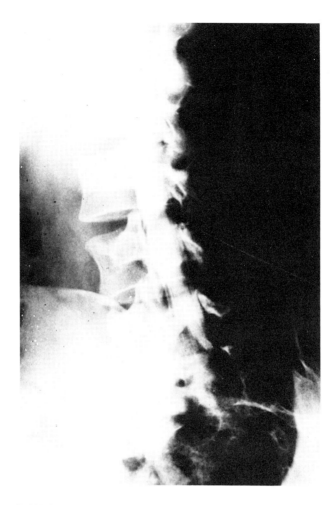

FIGURE 1. Lumbar myelogram with water-soluble contrast medium (Kontrast U Leo® 20%) shows the nerves of the cauda equina
separately in the oblique projection. A compression of a nerve is seen
at L₄ to L₅ level by a small lateral disk herniation. The disk protrusion
was not disclosed on a previous myelogram performed with insoluble
contrast medium (Myodil®).

its content is dissolved, because the air bubbles will delay the preparation of the solution. The solution in the vial should be used the same day when prepared, and if a
certain amount of the solution remains after the examination, it has to be discarded.[35]

The dose of Metrizamide® for myelography varies and should be determined depending upon the obesity of the patient, age, and the region to be examined.[12-14]
The amount of the contrast material injected into the subarachnoid space is usually
10 cc in the concentration of 170 mg I/mℓ. Some investigators have applied larger
quantities of contrast medium solutions in higher concentration.[11,17,25,27] It should be
pointed out that the total dose of 15 mℓ of 200 mg I/mℓ, or 10 mℓ of 300 mg I/mℓ
ought not to be exceeded. According to the experience of some authors, Metrizamide®
is the only water-soluble contrast medium that is well tolerated by children, and can
be safely used in pediatric radiology.[19-21] The recommended dose of the contrast medium for infants and children should not exceed 0.06 g of iodine per killogram body
weight.[19-21] Moreover, the estimated dose of Metrizamide® to be injected into the
subarachnoid space in children was calculated also in relation to the brain weight be-

cause of the possibility of serious complications that may be provoked if the contrast medium is distributed over the brain surface.[20] The introduction of Metrizamide® to pediatric radiology made myelography simpler and faster for the following reasons: general anesthesia is usually not necessary; the needle can be removed immediately after the injection of the contrast material that is not recovered; and the radiation dose is considerably reduced.[19-22]

For the lumbar puncture, a 3.5-in. long 22-gauge needle is used. The patient is in an upright, seated position on the fluoroscopic table. We have not applied the lateral decubitus with the cephalad 30° elevated table because of its tendency to be often the cause of epi-arachnoid injections of the contrast medium. In the sitting position of the patient with his back arched dorsally, it is simple to perform the puncture, mostly at the L_3 to L_4 level, for the reason of the elevated spinal fluid pressure and distended subarachnoid space. In children, however, the decubitus position may prove necessary and a shorter needle should be used. The advantage of the decubitus posture is the possibility to visualize, on the TV screen, the instillation of the contrast medium into the subarachnoid space. The puncture of the lumbar region is performed under sterile conditions, the needle is inserted precisely in the midline and directed ventrally and slightly in the cephalad direction. The elastic resistance of the dura is well felt, and after the perforation of the meninges, a free flow of CSF will occur. At this point the needle is attached to a plastic tube connected with the syringe. Some investigators will carry out the Queckenstedt test and manometric readings before the injection of the contrast medium. About 5 to 6 cc of CSF is removed for laboratory examination before the injection of the contrast medium begins. After the injection of Metrizamide® and the removal of the needle, the patient is placed in a prone position on the fluoroscopy table. The table is elevated for about 45° to bring the patient's head above the level of the lumbar region. Under the control of fluoroscopy, spot films are exposed in the prone and oblique positions of the lumbar area. After the fluoroscopic evaluation of the lumbar region, standard exposures are obtained in the anteroposterior, cross-table lateral, and both oblique projections. In order to clearly demonstrate the nerve root sleeves in the lumbar area, a lateral decubitus can be added to the standard exposures. In the course of the examination of the lumbo-sacral region, the patient has to be comfortably supported by the footstep attached to the table. Following the evaluation of the lower lumbar area, the table can be brought into a more horizontal position to demonstrate the upper lumbar and lower thoracic levels. The conus medullaris and the nerves forming the cauda equina are clearly visualized on Metrizamide® myelograms (Figure 2).[16,18]

For the examination of the *thoracic region,* a higher concentration of Metrizamide® is advised by some investigators. The average dose should be about 2.7 g of iodine or 200 to 250 mg I/mℓ[11,23,24] Different myelographic techniques have been described for the exploration of the thoracic region.[11,24-27] With some investigators, the cranial descent of the contrast medium, by turning the patient on his side, is a preferable technique. A gradual and slow tilting of the table for about 10° head down is performed under fluoroscopic control combined with spot radiography. In the prone position of the patient, the flow of the contrast medium can be rather fast and therefore this position is disadvantageous.[11] During the thoracic descent of the contrast medium, the head lies in a posterior flexion. It is essential to avoid the penetration of the contrast medium into the upper cervical subarachnoid space and the base of the skull. Following spot radiography under fluoroscopic control of the dorsal region, standard (cross-table lateral with a horizontal beam, posteroanterior, lateral decubitus, and oblique) radiographs are obtained.

As the contrast medium moves into the thoracic area, a progressive dilution occurs.

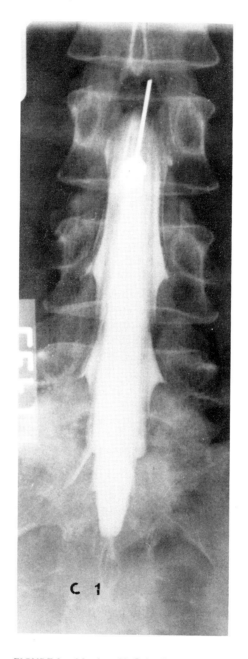

FIGURE 2.   Metrizamide® lumbar myelogram
in the prone anteroposterior position delineates
the nerves of the cauda equina with the meningeal sleeves.

Subsequently, the quality of myelograms may decline because the radiopacity of the
contrast medium becomes lower, and the detection of pathologic processes can be more
difficult.[11,24]

   The examination of the *cervical subarachnoid space* by means of Metrizamide® can
be achieved in several ways. The contrast medium can be injected either into the lumbar subarachnoid space or the cervical subarachnoid space using the lateral cervical
approach, or into the cisterna magna following the suboccipital puncture.[27,31] A higher

concentration of the contrast medium up to 300 mg I/ml is recommended if the contrast medium is injected into the lumbar or lateral cervical areas. If the suboccipital technique is employed, the amount of Metrizamide® solution should not exceed 5 ml of 300 mg I/ml.[28,32,33]

The examination of the cervical region includes spot radiographs under the control of fluoroscopy in anteroposterior and oblique positions, followed by standard cross-table lateral, "swimmer's", anteroposterior, and oblique projections. The patient's head is placed in the posterior flexion (extension) to prevent the flow of the contrast medium into the subarachnoid space of the skull.[29,30] Other projections can be used if deemed necessary. If the contrast medium is injected into the lumbar subarachnoid space, the examination of the cervical area is carried out first in order to avoid dilution.[29] Some investigators prefer the contrast medium to flow into the cervical region with the patient in the lateral decubitus.[30] Later in the course of the examination, the patient is turned to the opposite side so that a complete outlining of the spinal cord and nerve roots can be achieved. The exploration of the cervical area with Metrizamide® is simpler due to the fact that there is no fragmentation as it occurs with oily contrast media, and, in the presence of a complete block, the contrast medium does not augment the compression of the spinal cord and it is absorbed in a short period of time. The radiographic technique applied to the cervical area should produce radiographs of high quality to be able to outline the contrast medium in the cervical subarachnoid space.[34] Following the investigation of the cervical region, it is advisable to obtain a radiograph of the skull.

After Metrizamide® myelography, the patient ought to remain in bed for 24 hr with his head elevated. The bed can be raised for about 15 to 20°. Further on, the patient should be closely supervised during this period because of the possibility of seizures, especially in the first 8 to 10 hr. If the contrast medium escaped into the skull, it is recommended to administer intramuscularly 10 mg of diazepam (Valium®). Depending upon the situation, diazepam can be also used by an intravenous route.[35,36]

A complete elimination of Metrizamide® from the CSF makes myelography more tolerable to the patient, and technically much easier to carry out. The overall quality of radiographs following the subarachnoid injection of Metrizamide® is generally good for the lumbar region, in our experience. The delineation of the nerve roots in the lumbar area is better obtained, by far, by Metrizamide® than with oily contrast agents. A higher dilution of Metrizamide® can cause a decline of quality of cervical and thoracic myelograms.

REFERENCES

1. Epstein, B. S., *The Spine,* 4th ed., Lea & Febiger, Philadelphia, 1976, 92.
2. Cautico, W., Gannon, W., and Samouhos, E., A needle designed for myelography *J. Neurosurg.,* 28, 87, 1968.
3. Chynn, Y. K., Painless myelography: introduction of a new aspiration cannula and review of 541 consecutive studies, *Radiology,* 109, 361, 1973.
4. Shapiro, R., *Myelography,* 3rd ed., Year Book Medical Publishers, Chicago, 1975, chaps. 2, 4.
5. Haverling, M., Transsacral puncture of the arachnoidal sac, *Acta Radiol. Diagn.,* 12, 1, 1972.
6. Kelly, D. L. and Alexander, E., Jr., Lateral cervical puncture for myelography, *J. Neurosurg.,* 29, 106, 1968.
7. Mullan, S., Harper, P. V., Hekmatpanak, J., Torres, H., and Dobbin, G., Percutaneous interruption of spinal-pain tracts by means of a strontium needle, *J. Neurosurg.,* 20, 931, 1963.

8. **Salmon, J. H.,** Transventricular spinal myelography in the infant, *Radiology,* 91, 104, 1968.

9. **Taveras, J. M. and Wood, E. H.,** *Diagnostic Neuroradiology,* Vol. 2 (Part 7) 2nd ed., Williams & Wilkins, Baltimore, 1976, 1100.

10. **Skalpe, T. O. and Amundsen, P.,** Lumbar radiculography with Metrizamide. A nonionic water-soluble contrast medium, *Radiology,* 115, 91, 1975.

11. **Grainger, R. G., Kendall, B. E., and Wylle, J. G.,** Lumbar myelography with Metrizamide — a new nonionic contrast medium, *Br. J. Radiol.,* 49, 996, 1976.

12. **Dugstad, G. and Eldevik, P.,** Lumbar myelography, *Acta Radiol. Diagn.,* Suppl. 355, 17, 1977.

13. **Hekster, R. E. M., Prins, H. J., and Pennings-Braun, A. G. M.,** Lumbar myelography with Metrizamide, *Acta Radiol.,* Suppl. 355, 38, 1977.

14. **Oberson, R. and Azam, F.,** La radiculo-myélographie à L'Amipaque, *Med. Hyg.,* 35, 2485, 1977.

15. **Sortland, O., Lundervold, A., Svare, A., Hauglie-Hanssen, E.,** Metrizamide in radiography of the central nervous system, *Acta Radiol.,* Suppl. 347, 477, 1975.

16. **Sortland, O., Magnaes, B., and Hauge, T.,** Functional myelography with Metrizamide in the diagnosis of lumbar spinal stenosis, *Acta Radiol. Diagn.,* Suppl. 355, 42, 1977.

17. **Grainger, R. G.,** Technique of lumbar myelography with Metrizamide, *Acta Radiol. Diagn.,* Suppl. 355, 31, 1977.

18. **Skalpe, I. O., Torbergsen, T., Amudsen, P., and Presthus, J.,** Lumbar myelography with Metrizamide, *Acta Radiol. Diagn., Suppl.* 335, 367, 1973.

19. **Barry, J. F., Derek, C. Harwood-Nash, M. B., Fitz, C. R., Byrd, S. E., and Boldt, D. W.,** Metrizamide in pediatric myelography, *Neuroradiology,* 124, 409, 1977.

20. **Sortland, O. and Hovind, K.,** Myelography with Metrizamide in children, *Acta Radiol. Diagn.,* Suppl. 355, 211, 1977.

21. **Hugosson, C., Hindmarsh, T., and Bergstrom, K.,** Myelography with Metrizamide in infants and children, *Acta Radiol. Diagn.,* Suppl. 355, 193, 1977.

22. **Hugosson, C., Berstrand, G., and Hindmarsh, T.,** Thoraco-lumbar myelography in infants and children with a new water-soluble contrast medium, *Ann. Radiol.,* 20, 1, 1977.

23. **Valk, J.,** Thoracic myelography with Metrizamide, *Acta Radiol. Diagn.,* Suppl. 355, 77, 1977.

24. **Skalpe, I. O. and Sortland, O.,** Thoracic myelography with Metrizamide. Technical and diagnostic aspects, *Acta Radiol. Diagn.,* Suppl. 355, 57, 1977.

25. **Cronquist, S.,** Thoracic myelography with Metrizamide, *Acta Radiol. Diagn.,* Suppl. 355, 65, 1977.

26. **Hindmarsh, T.,** Myelography with the non-ionic water-soluble contrast medium Metrizamide, *Acta Radiol.,* 16, 417, 1975.

27. **Skalpe, I. O. and Amundsen, P.,** Thoracic and cervical myelography with Metrizamide. Clinical experiences with a water-soluble, non-ionic contrast medium, *Radiology,* 116, 101, 1975.

28. **Gonsette, R. E.,** Cervical myelography with Metrizamide by suboccipital puncture, *Acta Radiol. Diagn.,* Suppl. 355, 121, 1977.

29. **Sortland, O.,** Cervical myelography with Metrizamide using lumbar injection, *Acta Radiol. Diagn.,* Suppl. 355, 141, 1977.

30. **Hindmarsh, T.,** Metrizamide in selective cervical myelography, *Acta Radiol. Diagn.,* Suppl. 355, 127, 1977.

31. **Amundsen, P. and Skalpe, T. O.,** Cervical myelography with a water-soluble contrast medium (Metrizamide). A preliminary clinical report with special reference to technical aspects, *Neuroradiology,* 8, 209, 1975.

32. **Amundsen, P.,** Metrizamide in cervical myelography. Survey and present state, *Acta Radiol. Diagn.,* Suppl. 355, 85, 1977.

33. **Peters, F. L. M.,** Myelography with Metrizamide, *Radiol. Clin.,* 46, 203, 1977.

34. **Sortland, O. and Skalpe, T. O.,** Cervical myelography by lateral cervical and lumbar injection of Metrizamide. A comparison, *Acta Radiol. Diagn.,* Suppl. 355, 154, 1977.

35. Introduction, Metrizamide, *Acta Radiol. Diagn.,* Suppl. 335, 1973.

36. Introduction, Metrizamide, *Acta Radiol. Diagn.,* Suppl. 355, 1975.

Chapter 6

COMPLICATIONS RELATED TO POSITIVE CONTRAST MYELOGRAPHY

Complications related to myelography with opaque contrast media can be associated with: intrathecal action of the contrast medium; puncture of the subarachnoid space; myelographic technique; introduction of infection; and different medications used in conjunction with myelography. Some of these complications may have an acute onset, some, however, will appear in an insidious way with a chronic course.

Since their introduction, radiopaque *insoluble contrast media* have been recognized as possible sources of changes affecting the meninges and the nervous tissue.[1,2,5-7,21,39] These contrast agents act mainly in two ways: as foreign bodies that remain for an undetermined period of time in the subarachnoid space, and through the iodine fraction of their chemical structures. Possibly, some other chemical components in their structure may have an additional impact. It was postulated that Pantopaque® (Myodil®, Éthiodane®) could be absorbed after a certain period of time, and different measurements were used to determine more precisely the rate of its absorption. These experimental and clinical studies showed little practical value because the absorption of such contrast media proved to be very slow and unpredictable. Furthermore, the determination of the rate of absorption on radiographs, obtained at different intervals after myelography, was not an objective procedure. The diminishing radiopacity due to the absorption of iodine did not imply necessarily that other chemical components of the contrast agent were absorbed. In any case, the absorption of Pantopaque® or Lipiodol®, and of a number of similar compounds, was very slow, as observed by investigators.[1,2,8,10-13,15,16] To prevent a more prolonged, undesirable action of these contrast agents, their removal from the subarachnoid space has been recommended and practiced in some institutions.

The meningeal response to the presence of insoluble contrast medium was reflected by the spinal fluid changes that occurred as acute.[4,6] This prompt reaction was manifested by the rise of the white blood cells and protein in the spinal fluid. In the early Fifties, we carried out upon every procedure, analyses of the CSF, obtained under sterile conditions before and after instillation of the contrast medium (Myodil®). Following the instillation of the insoluble contrast medium, a reaction occurred which was detected in the second sample of the spinal fluid collected after myelography. Samples of the spinal fluid obtained at different intervals after myelography from some patients who for clinical reasons had to be repunctured, showed that the increase in the white cells and protein had been progressing for a period of time. Approximately after 5 to 7 days, it appeared that these reactive changes had the tendency to decrease, although in 12 patients they were still present 10 to 15 days after myelography. The first sample of the spinal fluid collected before the injection of the contrast medium did not reveal the presence of cells or protein in patients who did not have a complete or partial obstruction of the subarachnoid space. Aerobic and anaerobic cultures of the spinal fluid recovered before and after the installation of the contrast medium were negative.

After the subarachnoid instillation of insoluble contrast media an increase in protein with a variable number of lymphocytes, monocytes, and plasma cells with a smaller number of polymorphonuclear cells was found also by other investigators.[10,34,51] Many experimental and clinical studies were dedicated to the question of acute meningeal reactions following the injection of opaque contrast media.[17] The variability of reactions to Pantopaque® in different patients was connected to the tolerance of iodine, which varied. Variable degrees of aseptic meningitis in experimental studies with animals was similar to the variations in the clinical setting, which points to the possibility that the aseptic meningitis could be due to the differences in sensitivity towards iodine. The clinical study conducted by Luce on two patients, showed that 9 days in the first case following the skin test and myelography, and 30 days in the second case after these procedures, flare-ups occurred at the sites of intradermal tests. The signs of acute meningitis coincided with the flare-up of the skin reaction in both cases; both patients, however, showed a rapid subsidence of meningeal signs and a slower disappearance of skin reaction. It appears, according to this study, that the hypersensitivity to Pantopaque® was produced either by the intradermal injection, or by the subarachnoid instillation of the contrast agent, and possibly by both mechanisms. The preliminary skin test could be considered as a sensitizing medium.[28-30] The positive skin reactions to Pantopaque®, of immediate and delayed type, led some authors to the conclusion that simultaneous use of Pantopaque® for skin testing and for myelography was contraindicated.[28,29] Some experimental and clinical studies carried out in the Fifties and Sixties suggested that the irritating properties of Pantopaque® might be even more severe if the compound broke into small particles and was mixed with blood. It was postulated that blood might act as an emulsifying medium to disperse the chemical into small droplets.[10,20,25] Other studies, however, could not establish an amplified reaction of the meninges if the blood was mixed with ethyl-iodophenylundecanoate.[20,32] Certain investigators demonstrated that acute arachnoiditis caused by the contrast agent could be suppressed if corticosteroids were given intrathecally in combination with the contrast medium, or if injected parenterally.[19,31] Experiments done on animals indicated that the clinical signs such as hyperreflexia or ataxia corresponded to the severity of leptomeningitis induced by the intrathecal injection of opaque insoluble contrast media. The glucose values in the CSF following the injection of the contrast medium were below normal ranges, and the predominant cell type in the meningeal exudate was mononuclear.[20,24] The response of the leptomeninges in studied animals to the presence of insoluble contrast media developed rapidly, peaked in 5 days, and subsided after a period of time.[20,22] It should be noted here that an increase in cells in the spinal fluid and an elevation of temperature with or without headache may occur after lumbar or suboccipital punctures without injection of opaque media or other compounds.[18,42,43]

Prolonged elevation of the serum protein-bound iodine was established following myelography with ethyl-iodophenylundecanoate (Myodil®, Pantopaque®) for intervals varying between 2 and 16 years.[35-37] Possible hazards to health due to this protein-bound iodine found after myelography, such as thyreotoxicosis in adults with nodular goiter and congenital myxedema in the infants of affected mothers, were reported by some authors.[36,37]

Chronic leptomeningitis following myelography with insoluble and soluble contrast media refers mainly to localized or diffuse meningeal *adhesions*.[27] Some difficulties can be encountered in the process of establishing the presence of postmyelographic chronic arachnoiditis. In the clinical setting, the presence and extension of arachnoiditis is evaluated on the basis of the second, or eventually third myelographic study. A large number of these patients who come for the second myelography were operated upon in the period between the first and second examination of the subarachnoid space.[48,49] Therefore, it is often difficult to discern arachnoiditis caused by surgical treatment from the one that can be attributed to the impact of contrast media.[33,38,40,41,46,47,50,76,78] It is equally difficult to estimate the number of cases with postmyelographic arachnoiditis and to compare to the total number of myelographies performed with opaque contrast agents. Relatively few patients come for the second myelography, on the basis of which such determination can be reached. In addition, the interpretation of myelographic signs of arachnoiditis is subjective, except in advanced cases, and the congenital anatomic variations of the shape and size of the subarachnoid space can also be the cause of errors. In a study carried out in 1965 and 1967, we used gas myelography as a method for the evaluation of the subarachnoid space following myelography with opaque contrast media. The intensity of the late postmyelographic changes varied, and the results of this study suggested that the adhesions were less evident if the contrast medium was removed after the injection. The fixation of a larger mass or small drops of insoluble contrast media to the arachnoid occurred more often if the contrast medium was not removed. The absorption rate of this fixed contrast medium varied considerably from patient to patient (Figure 1 and 2).[7]

Detailed descriptions of postmyelographic leptomeningeal adhesions were written about by many authors on the basis of radiologic, experimental, and clinical observations.[23,24,46] Pathologic, surgical, and radiologic correlative studies in case of arachnoid adhesions are rare. The interpretation of the radiologic appearance of adhesions is thus based mostly on experimental work and on radiographic changes of the intrathecal distribution of the contrast medium, and the size and shape of the subarachnoid space. Experimentally, it is possible to produce arachnoiditis leading to adhesions by intracisternal injection of Pantopaque® in dogs. Adhesions can cause hydrocephalus and myelomalacia with disseminated cavitations in the cervical and thoracic regions of the spinal cord. It is assumed that the cavitations may be the sequence of vascular occlusions, or ischemia resulting from the compression of the meningeal blood vessels by fibrosis. The focal necrotic areas deriving from such ischemia were located mostly at the junction of the white and grey matter in the posterior portion of the spinal cord.[3,23] Experimental studies with large amounts of Pantopaque® injected into the subarachnoid space of monkeys showed that the retention of this contrast medium was always associated with a certain degree of arachnoid reaction. If the contrast medium was mixed with blood intrathecally, a more severe type of chronic arachnoiditis was provoked in some animals.[10,18,28,40,41] Mason and Raof estimate that the diffused aseptic meningitis is caused by hypersensitivity to Pantopaque®, and that the death in one of their patients following myelography was caused by the compression of the brain stem. The subarachnoid space in this reported case was obliterated with a membrane 1- to 10-mm thick.[5] According to Mason and Raof, a small percentage of people are hypersensitive to Pantopaque® and in those who are, an intrathecal instillation of any quantity can cause a severe meningeal reaction with possible catastrophic results.[5] For example, cases of diffused aseptic meningitis were reported occuring after myelography and causing increased intracranial pressure and internal hydrocephalus, sometimes with a fatal outcome.[9] In 1960, we had a patient who developed transient diplopia and nystagmus following myelography with Myodil® that was not removed. About 3 cc of Myodil® were injected. A few drops of the contrast medium penetrated into the region of the chiasmatic cistern, which were later disclosed on radiographs and tomograms of the skull. They remained fixed in the same position for approximately 14 months, diminishing, however, in size. The ocular clinical signs disappeared completely about 2 months after myelography. Using the technique of small quantities of the contrast medium (Myodil®, Éthiodane®) that would not be removed following myelography, we observed, on postmyelographic radiographs of the spine, the fragmentation and fixation of the contrast medium in the subarachnoid space (Figure 3). According to other studies and our personal experience, the follow up radiographs demonstrated signs of chronic leptomeningeal changes in the lumbosacral area in approximately 10 to 15% of reexamined patients in whom the contrast medium was not removed after myelography.[7,11-13] In patients with two or more myelographies and

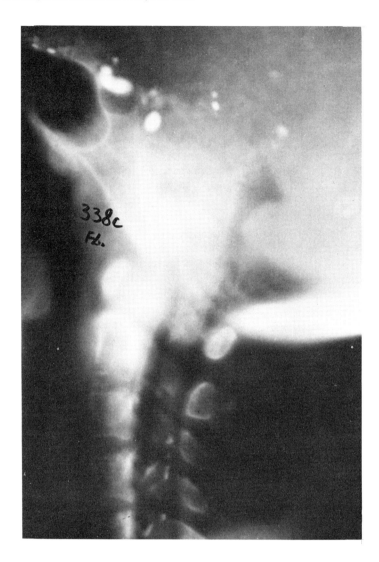

FIGURE 1.   A 37-year-old male patient previously had had myelographies
with positive insoluble contrast media because of a lumbar disk disease. This
time he was admitted with neck pain and signs of myelopathy. Gas myelography revealed fixed drops of a contrast medium in the cervical and thoracic
regions. Cisterna pontis could not be filled with oxygen. The fourth ventricle
and the cisterna cerebello-medullaris are clearly outlined by gas. Smaller and
larger drops of a contrast medium are seen in the area of cisterna chiasmatica, ambiens, interpeduncularis, and fossae Sylvii. These myelographic findings were interpreted as signs of diffuse arachnoid adhesions involving some
areas of the subarachnoid space in the skull.

incomplete removal of Pantopaque®, adhesive arachnoiditis was demonstrated at
laminectomy with a rope-like mass of nerve roots and cystic formations.[12] In addition,
a complete block of the subarachnoid space following myelography was described in
literature and it was established at surgery that it was due to the formation of inflammatory lipoid granuloma.[26]

   The serious, incapacitating, late complications following myelography with insoluble opaque media, described in literature, are relatively rare in percentage if compared

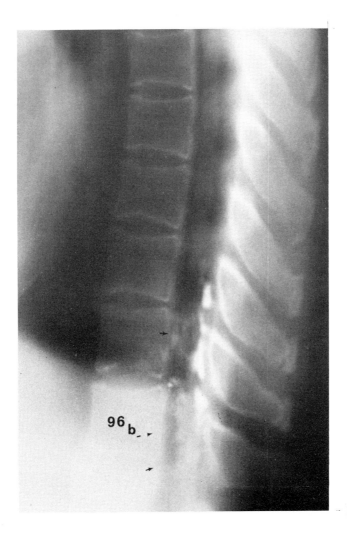

A

FIGURE 2 (A). Gas myelogram of this 42-year-old female patient
discloses an involvement of the lower thoracic spinal cord in thick
meningeal adhesions. In the region of the lumbar enlargement and
conus the spinal cord is not visible. The fixed streaks of the opaque
insoluble contrast can be seen (arrows). (B, C) In the thoracic region
the sagittal diameter of the clearly demarcated spinal cord is reduced.
This patient previously had had myelography with insoluble positive
contrast medium. The findings on the gas myelograms indicated that
the distal end of the spinal cord was embedded and compressed in
meningeal adhesions resulting in a diffuse spinal cord atrophy.

with the total number of myelographies performed with such contrast agents. A pru-
dent approach would be to remove the contrast medium following myelography (although opinions differ concerning this matter) and to reconsider the instillation of the
insoluble contrast agent in the presence of arachnoid hemorrhage of any origin.

Clinical signs that can be related to the irritative effect of insoluble contrast medium
on meninges causing a certain degree of morbidity in postmyelography patients are
diverse and vary greatly in intensity. Probably, the most common signs are backache

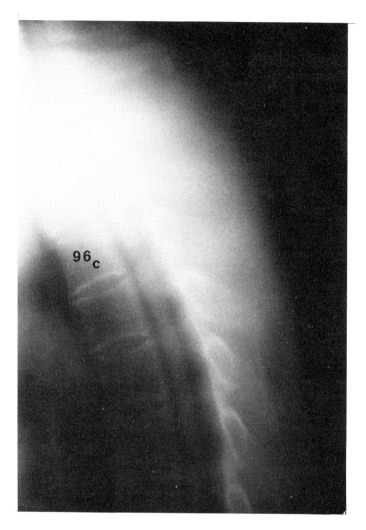

FIGURE 2B

and headache. The *backache*, which is common, is mostly localized, but it may extend into the leg and can be associated with muscle cramps or spasms. Some patients complain of an increase of exacerbation of the pain that was present prior to myelography. It was noted that the back pain could be more intense if a larger quantity of the insoluble contrast medium was used and left in the subarachnoid space following myelography.[43]

According to some clinical studies, *headache* following myelography occurred in about 29 to 46% of cases, and was comparable to the type of headache that developed after the lumbar puncture and removal of a large quantity of the CSF.[43,44] Since the introduction of the lumbar puncture by Quincke in 1891, headache became a well recognized complication of this procedure ("post-punktioneller Meningismus", Quincke).[45] Numerous theories have been proposed to explain its origin. Headache does occur following myelographies but, equally, it can originate from the lumbar puncture and thus, it is difficult to determine which of the two is the cause. If the contrast medium is fragmented, its removal following myelography is linked to the withdrawal of a considerable amount of the CSF that can aggravate the headache. Some investigators noted a more severe headache if a larger needle was used for the

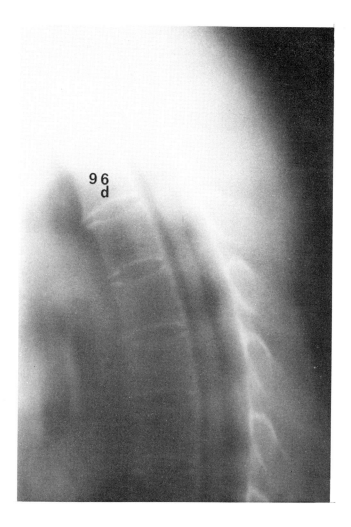

FIGURE 2C

puncture of the subarachnoid space (18 gauge).[18,43,92] In our experience, there was little difference in the severity of the headache when we used either a 22- or 18-gauge needle for the lumbar puncture, but there was, however, a difference if the technique was not adequate. If the needle is not inserted accurately into the subarachnoid space, it will damage the meninges and open a rather large hole in the dura through which the leakage of the spinal fluid will penetrate into the epidural space and cause the post-spinal puncture headache.[95] The spinal fluid will leak sometimes abundantly into the epidural space. This phenomenon was documented by the intrathecal injection of radionucleides in the region of cisterna magna. A high isotopic activity over the lumbar area following the descent of the radionucleide was recorded in the region of the extradural space.[13,44,70,95] Further on, incapacitating persistent headaches following myelographies were reported and treated by surgical repair of the needle hole. After surgery, a complete cure of the headache ensued.[44] It appears that an intrathecal instillation of methylprednisolone acetate (Depo-Medrol®) can be effective in preventing the headache.[18]

Following myelography, neck stiffness, nausea, vomiting, giddiness, cranial nerve palsy (third and fifth nerves), nystagmus, retention of urine, increased body tempera-

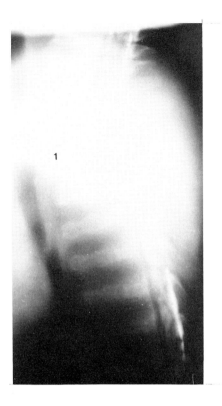
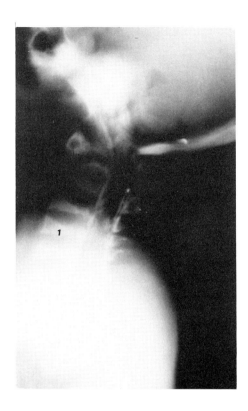

A   B

FIGURE 3(A). A four-year-old boy with congenital atlanto-axial dislocation had positive contrast myelography. The contrast was not removed. Approximately 1 year later gas myelography was performed. Gas myelogram demonstrates drops and streaks of fixed opaque contrast medium in the thoracic area dorsal to the spinal cord. (B) The cervical spinal cord is encompassed by gas and fixed opaque contrast. The double contrast myelogram was obtained due to the presence of the trapped opaque contrast medium. A drop of the contrast is seen fixed at the posterior wall of the cisterna magna. At surgery, meningeal adhesions were found in the upper cervical region. The patient was operated on in order to correct the atlanto-axial dislocation.

ture, sensory changes, a state of shock, ileus, etc. were also described.[5,11,43] The incident of minor and major complaints after myelography is relatively high, which indicates that this diagnostic procedure involves a significant risk of morbidity and should not be considered as a routine type of examination.[43]

Meningitis resulting from an introduction of different microorganisms in the course of puncture of the subarachnoid space was reported by several authors.[52,53] In an extensive review, Stanley described 14 cases of meningitis caused by *Bacillus pyocyaneus* introduced into the subarachnoid space in the course of the diagnostic lumbar puncture.[52] Cases of meningitis were described following lumbar punctures in connection with spinal anesthesia, and instillation of an opaque medium for myelography.[53] The cause of postmyelographic meningitis was found to be *Pseudomonas aeruginosa,* a normal inhabitant of the skin and gastrointestinal tract.

Complications related to the instillation of insoluble opaque contrast media can be different in nature. These contrast agents may inadvertently enter the venous system during lumbar myelography. The intravasation of Pantopaque® and similar compounds was well documented in 22 cases by different authors.[54-61] In 1945, Hinkel gave a detailed description of Pantopaque® intravasation following lumbar subarachnoid instillation.[61] The contrast medium did not immediately enter the veins and the spinal fluid was clear. Four minutes after the injection following cough and strain, the contrast medium was observed on fluoroscopy to leave the subarachnoid space through multiple channels representing the veins. The intravasation of Pantopaque® was fast, and in 30 sec it was seen in the inferior vena cava and different tributary veins. In this case, apparently, the cough was the factor that caused the rise in the CSF pressure. Coughing, sneezing, and other straining may increase the pressure of the spinal fluid many times the pressure in the abdominal veins, especially if the patient is in a prone position.

Rich venous plexuses (the posterior internal and anterior internal plexus) drain the blood from the basivertebral veins, medulla, and meninges. They are situated between the dura and the bone, and are profusely linked by venous rings (retia venosa vertebrarum). Both plexuses communicate with the intravertebral veins and the lumbar and lateral sacral veins that drain into the inferior vena cava. The needle tip, in the course of the lumbar puncture, can lacerate one or more of the veins that form the rich network encompassing the cord and subarachnoid space. The contrast material under these circumstances, especially if the spinal fluid pressure is raised, could intravasate into the systemic venous circulation and its emboli can be trapped in the capillary system of the lungs. Cough, pain, discomfort in the chest, tachycardia, fever, and occasionally small hemoptysis are the main clinical signs of multiple Pantopaque® emboli, and they are usually transient. The radiographic demonstration of the emboli depends, as it appears, on the quantity of Pantopaque® absorbed by the venous system. According to some investigators, the amount of over 7.5 cc is necessary to produce the radiographic evidence of lung embolization.[59] It was noted that the radiographic changes related to the Pantopaque® emboli tend to lodge chiefly in the anterior portion of the chest. This occurrence could be attributed to the effect of gravity. Radiologic pulmonary changes disappear within 24 hr, yet they can be detected 6 days after the intravasation.[59] In view of the possibility of Pantopaque® pulmonary embolism, some authors suggest that myelography be deferred temporarily if the spinal fluid appears bloody.[58,59] The intravasation of the opaque contrast medium during the instillation or removal has been described as complete or partial "sudden disappearance" of contrast medium.[58,62]

A spinal fluid-venous fistula was described as a possible additional mechanism through which an intravenous infusion of Pantopaque® can occur during myelography.[55] It has been demonstrated that opaque contrast media can easily flow from the subarachnoid space through the hole in the dura into the epidural space. The spinal fluid pressure in the prone position is approximately 160 to 200 mm H_2O, and the pressure in the epidural veins is lower, depending upon the phase of respiratory movements and straining of the patient. With the patient in the prone position, the flow of blood in the epidural veins is rapid and can also produce a suction effect, according to Venturi's law, which will further facilitate the passage of the fluid from the subarachnoid space into the venous channels with lower pressure. The mechanism of the CSF venous fistula indicates that a similar phenomenon can be the cause of headaches that follow the lumbar puncture. Theoretically, the CSF venous fistula can be the cause of prolonged intracranial hypotension.[55]

An instillation of the opaque insoluble contrast medium into the subdural or epidural spaces occurs much more often than intravasation. If the instillation is performed under fluoroscopy control, the characteristic signs of epidural spreading of the contrast medium can be recognized promptly and the injection stopped. With gentle suction, a small quantity of the contrast medium can sometimes be removed from the epidural space, yet it seems a better choice to remove the needle from the lumbar area and repeat the myelography about 2 weeks later. If such a delay is not possible because of clinical reasons, the injection of the contrast medium into the cervical or suboccipital areas should be considered. The injection of the contrast medium into the subdural space is not often recognized in the beginning of the instillation, especially if the examiner is not sufficiently experienced with myelographic techniques. As it is rather difficult to remove the contrast medium from the subdural space, persistent attempts should be avoided (Figure 4).

Injuries to the nerve filament are another common complication. The nerve can be partially lacerated during the attempts at lumbar puncture. A complete transection of the nerve filament and its suction through the needle may occur.[63,64] The removal of the contrast medium through a stylet with side holes and no end hole is safer than the utilization of needles or stylets with end holes. Puncture of a protruded disk, or different types of tumors, does occur rather often in the course of a myelographic procedure.[64,65,70]

Spinal epidural or subdural hematomas can furthermore complicate the lumbar puncture. They have been described following lumbar puncture in the patients with thrombocytopenia.[71] Although these types of complications are rare, they should be taken into consideration because of their fatal effect on the patient. The lower the platelet count, the more likely spinal hematoma is to complicate the lumbar puncture. A rapid dropping of the platelet count can take place when the spinal puncture is performed in patients who had the platelet count within the safe range. If myelography must be performed in patients with thrombocytopenia, platlets should be administered if the count is below 20,000, and the puncture of the subarachnoid space performed by an experienced investigator with a No. 22 needle. A careful observation of the patient is required after such myelography.

With patients in a prone position for a longer period of time, and especially with a tilted table head-down, *cardiovascular complications* can occur in the process of myelography. Cardiac arrest was described as the most serious problem, the genesis of which can be different.[68,69] The occurrence of *intraspinal epidermoids* was connected with lumbar puncture, disk puncture, or myelography.[66,67] Appearance of severe reflex *algodystrophy* and *coccygodynia* following myelography was described as an unusual complication of this procedure.[72,73]

Complications with the utilization of water-soluble contrast media, previously used, will be briefly discussed. Some of the side effects connected to the employment of these contrast agents were mentioned above. For over 10 years, we had used rather extensively a 20% buffered solution of monoiodomethane sulfonate sodium methiodol (Kontrast U® 20% Leo) which contains 10.4% by weight of organically bound iodine. It is a hypertonic solution, equivalent to a 5.1% solution of saline. This hyperbaric contrast medium was supposed to retain its radiopacity by displacing the spinal fluid in the subarachnoid space rather than mixing with it.[74,75] Before the injection of the contrast medium, the spinal anesthesia was performed and the motor paralysis in both lower limbs with sensory paralysis at the groin level was achieved in approximately 10 min. The contrast medium in the quantity of 10 cc was injected at the site of the lumbar puncture, generally between L_4 and L_5, with an even, gentle pressure on the plunger of the syringe in order to diminish any turbulence and prevent the ascent of the hypertonic, hyperbaric contrast agent in the direction of the spinal cord. After the injection, the needle would be removed. In a series of cases, we did not remove the needle immediately but following the radiographic procedure. After the radiographs were obtained, we would collect about 2 cc of the spinal fluid from the spinal canal so that we could proceed with the second laboratory examination. The comparison of the laboratory findings between the first and second sample established a rather fast increase in cells and protein following the injection of the contrast medium.

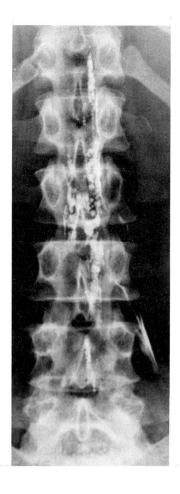

A

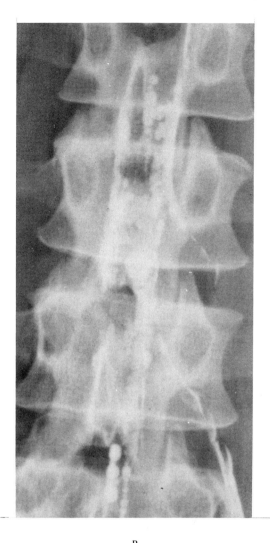

B

FIGURE 4. Standard radiographs of the lumbar spine disclosed the epidural and subdural spreading of the opaque contrast medium injected a few weeks earlier when, according to the patient, a myelography was performed.

An additional common complication was the decrease of blood pressure combined with more or less pronounced signs of shock. The drop of blood pressure was, in most instances, possible to control with repeated injection of ephedrine or similar medications, and administration of oxygen and I.V. saline. The next fairly common complication was the cramping pain in the back, perineum, and in the lower extremities, which could be very intensive. It was assumed that this pain was provoked by the descent of the contrast medium into the sacral subarachnoid sac. Occasionally, it was possible to minimize the pain by placing the patient in the prone position. Other complications were reported including bladder and rectal paralysis, persistent sacral anesthesia, convulsions, partial paralysis, etc.[76-78] It was accepted to avoid the contrast agents of the sodium methiodal type in the event of scoliosis since it might enhance the ascent of the hypertonic, hyperbaric solution, especially if the patient was turned from one side to the other in the course of the radiographic procedure.

A number of excellent clinical and experimental studies were concerned with the side effects of sodium methiodal. On experimental animals, it was established that extensive meningeal cell infiltration with lymphocytes mainly, often extended throughout the length of the spinal cord. The cell infiltration of the spinal cord was mostly perivascular. Generalized muscle twitching and jerky extensor spasms of the limbs developed in rabbits after the suboccipital injection of 0.2 to 0.4 cc of 20% sodium methiodal, and 17 out of 39 rabbits died within 24 hr after the injection.[79] Experimentally, the fall of the blood pressure was attributed to the paralysis of the axons in the anterior nerve roots.[80,81] The acute swelling of the nerve cells caused by sodium methiodal was considered to be a characteristic feature of acute intoxication, and clinical complications were presumed possible due to this toxic action on the spinal cord and neurons.[22,82] Clinical and experimental observations suggest, as mentioned in the previous text, that the water-soluble contrast media are hyperosmolal in comparison with the CSF, and that the high osmotic gradient between the CSF and the neural elements is the factor that contributes to different clinical manifestations of toxicity.[14] It was demonstrated, besides, that the toxicity of water-soluble contrast media was related to their lipid solubility.[83,84] It is possible that the lumbar anesthesia used in conjunction with methiodal sodium myelography could have been in some cases a contributing factor to the development of postmyelographic adhesions.[85]

The supposition was that the introduction of methylglucamine iothalamate (Conray 60%®, Conray Meglumine 282®, Contrix 28®) and methylglucamine iocarmate (Dimer X®) would alleviate the unfavorable side effects of sodium methiodal. Experimental studies carried out with methylglucamine iothalamate and sodium methiodal suggested that both contrast media caused similar histologic changes in and around the spinal cord, but these alterations were more prominent following the administration of sodium methiodal.[98,110,112-114] Delayed and prolonged clonic spasm developed in rabbits following injection of 0.4 cc of methylglucamine iothalamate 30% into the suboccipital area. Of the 37 rabbits used for the experimental work, 7 died within 24 hr after the injection.[79]

Methylglucamine iothalamate and methylglucamine iocarmate proved less toxic and could be used without spinal anesthesia. Their utilization, however, was restricted mainly to the lumbosacral area. After the instillation of these contrast media, pleocytosis occurred in clinical and experimental settings. Other different clinical complications were attributed to these two contrast media, such as headache and vomiting, stiffness of the neck, increase in original pain, myoclonic spasms, hypotension, perasthesia, and arachnoid adhesions.[106-111] Headache is a common occurrence with all the three prevously used water-soluble contrast media.[82,116] Mycoclonic spasms can be controlled in most instances by intravenous injection of 10 mg of diazepam (Valium®).[81,87]

With the introduction of Metrizamide®, the number and intensity of side effects were sharply reduced. Comparative studies carried out with methylglucamine iothalamate (Conray®) and methylglucamine iocarmate, and Metrizamide® indicated that Metrizamide®, in clinical application, was less toxic than the two previously used contrast agents.[84,96,114,117] Metrizamide® is usually well tolerated if applied in lumbar myelography. Grand mal seizures and clonic convulsions are less frequent in our experience and according to extensive clinical observations.[86-91] Most authors agree that the most common complications following myelography with Metrizamide® are headaches that occurred in approximately 62%, and nausea and/or vomiting in 38% of cases.[86,87,94] The occurrence of these reactions is about the same with Metrizamide® as with meglumine iocarmate (Dimer X®).[93,97] Also, more common side effects of Metrizamide® myelography are back and leg pain, neck stiffness, and elevated body temperature.[86] Less common complications of Metrizamide® subarachnoid installation are paresthesias, dizziness or diplopia, skin rash, voiding difficulty, olfactory disturbances, diarrhea, photophobia, leg spasms, and agitation.[86,101] The frequency of adverse reactions attributed to Metrizamide® myelography varies from one study to another, depending upon the amount of contrast medium used, myelographic technique, pathologic processes, age of the patient, and other contributing factors such as general anesthesia or premedication. Complications linked to the intrathecal injection of Metrizamide® appear to be transient. Infiltration by white blood cells of the spinal cord, meninges, and nerve roots was found in about 20% of experimental animals after myelography.[79,84]

The application of Metrizamide® in the thoracic area did not provoke clonic-tonic convulsions, and EEG changes were seen in about 20% of patients.[91,96,99] Headache, nausea, and vomiting were more pronounced and happened more often when the contrast medium was moved into the thoracic region. The higher concentration of the contrast medium used for the evaluation of the thoracic spine might be the cause of these reactions. In a small number of cases, other complication were found related to thoracic myelography with Metrizamide® such as pain, paresthesias and numbness in the legs, increase in body temperature, confusion, areflexia, and psychotic and depressive signs.[86,100] These adverse reactions were transient.

The reactions to the cervical Metrizamide® myelography emerged as more pronounced. Epileptic seizures occurred, and were controlled by intravenous injection of diazepam (Valium®).[96,97,101] In addition, generalized spasms were described.[101] These complications were attributed to the higher concentration of the contrast medium and volumes used for the exploration of the cervical area and possible distribution of Metrizamide® over the cerebral cortex. Such type of complications stress the importance of careful fluoroscopic observation of the flow of Metrizamide® in the cervical region. It is important equally, to prevent the flow of Metrizamide® into the intracranial subarachnoid spaces, especially those covering the cortex of the brain.[101] It is advisable to obtain a radiograph of the skull after myelography to check whether the contrast medium has passed intracranially. If this should be the case, the patient has to be observed carefully for at least 24 hr. The EEG recordings made following cervical myelography showed changes in approximately 22% of patients.[96,103] Dizziness and pain were described in case of cervical Metrizamide® myelography, as well as mental reactions, transient in nature, and mental confusion associated with epileptic seizures.[101,102,115] In all probability, the adverse reactions following cervical myelography with Metrizamide® depend, to a certain degree, on the technique and experience of the investigator, and the amount and concentration of Metrizamide®. It seems probable that the route of injection, lumbar or suboccipital, might also have a certain effect.

On the basis of available experimental results and clinical experiences it looks, at present, as if Metrizamide® could be the least toxic water-soluble contrast medium. Metrizamide's® relatively low toxicity and reduced biologic and pharmacologic activity enables the usage of its higher concentration and thus the improvement of quality of radiographs. The concentration of Metrizamide® can vary, which is a considerable asset, depending on the needs of the examiner, and the age and clinical state of the patient. It is possible to perform with considerable ease the so-called functional myelography using Metrizamide®. In addition, Metrizamide® myelography is better facilitated since the removal of the contrast medium is not necessary and the needle is withdrawn from the subarachnoid space after injection. The filling of narrow subarachnoid spaces can be better achieved with Metrizamide® owing to its miscibility with the CSF, and its low viscosity. The density of Metrizamide® does not obscure the details on radiographs, and there is no fragmentation of the contrast medium. The protein bound iodine values in plasma are not influenced more than 2 to 3 weeks after the instillation of Metrizamide® into the subarachnoid space. Patients who might be hypersensitive to iodine-containing contrast agents should be given special attention if Metrizamide® is used. It is recommended to give to the patient as premedication corticosteroids or antihistamines to prevent undesirable side effects. However, these medications should not be mixed with Metrizamide. ®

Long-term sequelae of Metrizamide® myelography are difficult to evaluate because this contrast agent has not been used for a long enough period of time. Moreover, the evaluation of late changes are related to the same difficulties as with other contrast media. Histological examination of the human CNS, nerve roots, and meninges after intrathecal instillation of contrast media occurred only occasionally.[84] Clinical observations based on repeated myelographies using water-soluble contrast media such as sodium methiodal and meglumine iothalamate indicate the frequency of arachnoid adhesions established on radiographs. Apparently, the intensity of these findings was related to the concentration and the amount of contrast medium as well as the protein content of the CSF.[103-106,112-114] Concerning the utilization of Metrizamide® and the appearance of arachnoid adhesions, some experimental works indicated that these changes could take place, and that the increase in osmolarity alone does not produce arachnoiditis and adhesions. Clinical studies, however, do not support, at present, the theory that Metrizamide® can be the cause of radiographically apparent arachnoid adhesions as is the case with other water-soluble contrast media.[25,103-105] So far, available data do not indicate that the long term sequelae of Metrizamide® myelography are common.[86,108,113,117]

REFERENCES

1. **Lindblom, A. F.,** Effect of Lipiodol on the meninges, *Acta Radiol.,* 5, 129, 1926.
2. **Craig, W. McK.,** Use and abuse of iodized oil in the diagnosis of lesions of the spinal cord, *Surg. Gynecol. Obstet.,* 49, 17, 1929.
3. **McLaurin, R. L.,** Myelomelacia and multiple cavitations of spinal cord secondary to adhesive arachnoiditis, *Arch. Pathol.,* 57, 138, 1954.
4. **Ramsey, G. H.,** Iodinated organic compounds as contrast media for radiographic diagnosis, IV., *Radiology,* 43, 236, 1944.
5. **Mason, M. S. and Raof, J.,** Complications of Pantopaque myelography: case report and review, *J. Neurosurg.,* 19, 302, 1962.
6. **Markovich, A. W.,** Immediate and late effects of intrathecal injection of iodized oil, *JAMA,* 116, 2247, 1941.
7. **Bering, E. A., Jr.,** Notes on retention of Pantopaque in subarachnoid space, *Am. J. Surg.,* 80, 445, 1950.
8. **Peacher, W. G. and Robertson, R. C. L.,** Pantopaque myelography, *J. Neurosurg.,* 2, 220, 1945.
9. **Erickson, T. C. and Van Baaren, H. J.,** Late meningeal reaction of ethyliodophenylundecanoate used in myelography; report of case that terminated fatally, *JAMA,* 153, 636, 1953.
10. **Jaeger, R.,** Irritating effect of iodized vegetable oils on brain, spinal cord when divided into small particles, *Arch. Neurol. Psychiatry,* 64, 715, 1950.
11. **Davies, F. L.,** Effect of unabsorbed contrast media on the central nervous system, *Lancet,* 11, 747, 1956.
12. **Hurteau, E. F.,** Arachnoiditis following the use of iodized oil, *J. Bone J. Surg.,* 36, 393, 1954.
13. **Richtie, G. W. and Sinclair, D. J.,** Morbidity in post-myelography patients. A survey of 100 patients, *J. Can. Assoc. Radiol.,* 23, 278, 1972.

14. **Slatis, P.,** Hyperosmolarity of the cerebrospinal fluid as a cause of adhesive arachnoiditis in lumbar myelography, *Acta Radiol. Diagn.,* 15, 6, 629, 1974.
15. **French, J. D.,** Clinical manifestations of lumbar spinal arachnoiditis, *Surgery,* 20, 718, 1946.
16. **Mackay, R. P.,** Chronic adhesive spinal arachnoiditis, *JAMA,* 112, 802, 1939.
17. **Howland, W. J. and Curry, J. L.,** Experimental studies of Pantopaque arachnoiditis, *Radiology,* 87, 253, 1966.
18. **McLennan, J. E.,** Prevention of postmyelographic and postpneumoencephalographic headache by single dose intrathecal methylprednisolone acetate, *Headache,* 13, 39, 1971.
19. **Asbury, A, K.,** The inflammatory lesion in idiopathic polyneuritis, *Medicine,* 48, 173, 1969.
20. **Wilson, J. W.,** Acute leptomeningeal reaction to the subarachnoid injection of ethyliodophenylundecylate in dogs, *J. Am. Vet. Med. Assoc.,* 169, 415, 1976.
21. **Meacham, W. F. and Tolchin, S.,** The ependymal response to long-term intraventricular Pantopaque, *J. Neurol. Neurosurg. Psychiatr.,* 26, 559, 1963.
22. **Jakobsen, J. K.,** Clinical evaluation of a histologic examination of the side effects of myelographic contrast media, *Acta Radiol. Diagn.* 14, 638, 1973.
23. **Teng, P. and Paratheodorou, C.,** Myelographic findings in adhesive spinal arachnoiditis, *Br. J. Radiol.,* 40, 201, 1967.
24. **Smith, R. W. and Loeser, J. D.,** A myelographic variant in lumbar arachnoiditis, *J. Neurosurg.,* 36, 441, 1972.
25. **Irstam, L., Sundström, R., and Sigstedt, B.,** Lumbar myelography and adhesive arachnoiditis, *Acta Radiol. Diagn.,* 15, 356, 1974.
26. **Sarkisian, S. S.,** Spinal cord pseudotumor, *U.S. Armed Forces Med. J.,* 7, 1683, 1956.
27. **Tarlov, J. M.** Pantopaque meningitis disclosed at operation, *JAMA,* 129, 1014, 1945.
28. **Luce, J. C., Leith, W., and Burrage, W. S.,** Pantopaque meningitis due to hypersensitivity, *Radiology,* 57, 878, 1951.
29. **Jones, T. D. and Mote, J. R.,** Phases of foreign protein sensitization in human beings, *N. Engl. J. Med.,* 210, 120, 1934.
30. **Mackenzie, G. M. and Hanger, F. M., Jr.,** Allergic reactions to streptococcus antigens, *J. Immunol.,* 13, 41, 1927.
31. **Smith, J. K. and Ross, L.,** Steroid supression of meningeal inflammation caused by pantopaque, *J. Neurol.,* 9, 48, 1959.
32. **Fisher, R. L.,** An experimental evaluation of Pantopaque and other recently developed myelographic contrast media, *Radiology,* 85, 537, 1965.
33. **Wilson, J. W., Greene, H. J., and Leipold, H. W.,** Osseous metaplasia of the spinal dura mater in great dane, *J. Am. Vet. Med. Assoc.,* 167, 75, 1975.
34. **Peacher, W. G. and Robertson, R. C. H.,** Pantopaque myelography: results, comparison of contrast media, and spinal fluid reaction, *J. Neurosurg.,* 2, 220, 1945.
35. **White, A. G.,** Prolonged elevation of serum protein-bound iodine following myelography with Myodil, *Br. J. Radiol.,* 45, 21, 1972,
36. **Davis, P. J.,** Factors affecting the determination of serum protein-bound iodine, *Am. J. Med.,* 40, 918, 1966.
37. **Shapiro, R.,** The effect of maternal ingestion of iophenoxic acid on the serum protein-bound iodine on the progeny, *N. Engl. J. Med.,* 264, 378, 1961.
38. **Seaman, W. B., Marder, S. N., and Rosenbaum, H. E.,** The myelographic appearance of adhesive spinal arachnoiditis, *J. Neurosurg.,* 10, 145, 1953.
39. **Praestholm, J., Klee, J. G., and Klinken, L.,** Histological changes in the central nervous system following intraventricular administration of oil-soluble contrast media, *Radiology,* 119, 391, 1976.
40. **Bergeron, R.T., Rumbaugh, C. L., Fang, H., and Cravioto, H.,** Experimental Pantopaque arachnoiditis in the monkey, *Radiology,* 99, 95, 1971.
41. **Imielinski, L. and Chmielewski, J. M.,** Arachnoiditis adhesive intrachdiene à la suite de myelographies a l'Éthiodane (Pantopaque), *J. Radiol. Electrol.,* 52, 31, 1971.
42. **Taren, J. A.,** Unusual complication following pantopaque myelography, *J. Neurosurg.,* 17, 323, 1960.
43. **Sinclair, D. J. and Ritchie, G. W.,** Morbidity in post-myelogram patients — a survey of 100 patients, *J. Assoc. Can. Radiol.,* 23, 278, 1972.
44. **Gass, H., Goldstein, A. S., Ruskin, R., and Leopold, N. A.,** Chronic postmyelogram headache, *Arch. Neurol.,* 25, 169, 1971.
45. **Quincke, H.,** Die Lumbalpunktion des Hydrocephalus, *Berl. Klin. Wochenschr.,* 28, 965, 1891.
46. **Moseley, I.,** The oil myelogram after operation for lumbar disc lesions, *Clin. Radiol.,* 28, 267, 1977.
47. **Davidoff, L. M., Gass, H., and Grossman, J.,** Postoperative spinal adhesive arachnoiditis and recurrent spinal cord tumor, *J. Neurosurg.,* 4, 451, 1947.

48. Smolik, E. A. and Nash, F. P., Lumbar spinal arachnoiditis: a complication of the intervertebral disc operation, *Ann. Surg.*, 133, 490, 1951.
49. Turnbull, F., Postoperative inflammatory disease of lumbar disc, *J. Neurosurg.*, 10, 469, 1953.
50. Silver, M. L., Field, E. A., Silver, C. M., and Simon, S. D., The postoperative lumbar myelogram, *Radiology*, 72, 344, 1959.
51. David, J. R., Lymphocyte mediators and cellular hypersensitivity, *N. Engl. J. Med.*, 288, 143, 1973.
52. Stanley, M. M., Bacillus pyocyaneous infections, *Am. J. Med.*, 2, 253, 347, 1947.
53. Hobbs, M. L., Harley, J. B., and Love, B. F., Meningitis due to *pseudomonas aeruginosa* following myelography with pantopaque, *W. Va. Med. J.*, 53, 180, 1957.
54. Aspelin, P. and Lester, J., Pantopaque pulmonary embolism following myelography, *Neuroradiology*, 14, 43, 1977.
55. Lin, P. M. and Clarke, J., Spinal fluid-venous fistula: a mechanism for intravascular Pantopaque infusion during myelography, *J. Neurosurg.*, 41, 773, 1974.
56. Schultz, E. C. and Miller, J. H., Intravasation of opaque media during myelography, *J. Neurosurg.*, 18, 610, 1961.
57. Todd, M. E. and Gardner, W. J., Pantopaque intravasation (embolization) during myelography, *J. Neurosurg.*, 14, 230, 1957.
58. Ginsburg, L. B. and Skorneck, A. B., Pantopaque pulmonary embolism: a complication of myelography, *Am. J. Roentgenol.*, 73, 27, 1955.
59. Steinbach, H. L. and Hill, W. B., Pantopaque pulmonary embolism during myelography, *Radiology*, 56, 735, 1951.
60. Fullenlove, T. M., Venous intravasation during myelography, *Radiology*, 53, 410, 1949.
61. Hinkel, C. L., The entrance of Pantopaque into the venous system during myelography, *Am. J. Roentgenol.*, 54, 230, 1945.
62. Epstein, B. S. and Epstein, J. A., The cineroentgenographic observations of Pantopaque intravasation during myelography, *Am. J. Roentgenol.*, 94, 576, 1955.
63. Young, D. A. and Burney, R. E., II, Complication of myelography transsection and withdrawal of a nerve filament by the needle, *N. Engl. J. Med.*, 285, 156, 1971.
64. Everett, A. D., Lumbar puncture injuries, *Proc. R. Soc. Med.*, 35, 208, 1942.
65. Gellman, M., Injury to intravertebral discs during spinal puncture, *J. Bone J. Surg.*, 22, 980, 1940.
66. Manno, N. J., Uihlein, A., and Kernohan, J. W., Intraspinal epidermoids, *J. Neurosurg.*, 19, 754, 1962.
67. Boyd, H., Iatrogenic intraspinal epidermoid. Report of a case, *J. Neurosurg.*, 24, 105, 1966.
68. Cooper, D. R., Cardiac arrest on the myelographic tilt table, *JAMA*, 187, 674, 1964.
69. Zir, L. M., Carvalho, A. C., Harthorne, J. W., Colman, R. W., and Lees, R. S., Contrast agents, platelet aggregation and 14C-serotomine release, *N. Engl. J. Med.*, 291, 134, 1974.
70. Dripps, R. D. and Vandam, L. D., Hazards of lumbar puncture, *JAMA*, 147, 1118, 1951.
71. Edelson, R. N., Chernik, N. L., and Posner, J. B., Spinal subdural hematomas complicating lumbar puncture, *Arch. Neurol.*, 31, 134, 1974.
72. Miller, D. S., Post-myelographic coccygodynia, *Am. J. Proctol.*, 18, 292, 1967.
73. Morettin, L. B. and Wilson, McC., Severe reflex algodystrophy (Sudek's atrophy) as a complication of myelography: report of two cases, *Am. J. Roentgenol.*, 110, 156, 1970.
74. Arnell, S., Myelography with water-soluble contrast with special regard to the normal Roentgen picture, *Acta Radiol. Diagn.*, Suppl. 75, 1, 1948.
75. Lindblom, K., Lumbar myelography by Abrodil, *Acta Radiol. Diagn.*, 27, 1, 1946.
76. Lindblom, K., Complications of myelography by Abrodil, *Acta Radiol. Diagn.*, 28, 69, 1947.
77. Gund, A., Über eine komlikation bei Abrodil — Myelographie und ihre verhutung, *Wien. Med. Wochenschr.*, 105, 467, 1955.
78. Panter, K., Über komplikationen und gefahren bei der Abrodil — Myelographie, *Dtsch. Med. Wochenschr.*, 78, 937, 1953.
79. Praestholm, J. and Olgaard, K., Comparative histological investigation of sequelae of experimental myelography using sodium methiodal and meglumine iothalamate, *Neuroradiology*, 4, 14, 1972.
80. Praestholm, J. and Moller, S., Cardiovascular reactions to myelography with water soluble contrast media, *Neuroradiology*, 13, 195, 1977.
81. Allen, W. E., III, Van Gilder, J. C., and Collins, W. F., Evaluation of the neurotoxicity of water-soluble myelographic contrast agents by electrophysiological monitors, *Radiology*, 118, 89, 1976.
82. Peterson, H. O., The hazards of myelography, *Radiology*, 115, 237, 1975.
83. Levitan, H. and Rapoport, S. I., Contrast media. Quantitative criteria for designing compounds with low toxicity, *Acta Radiol. Diagn.*, 17, 81, 1976.
84. Praestholm, J., Experimental evaluation of water soluble contrast media for myelography, *Neuroradiology*, 13, 25, 1977.

85. **Winkelman, N. W., Gotten, N., and Scheibert, D.,** Localized adhesive spinal arachnoiditis, *Trans. Am. Neurol. Assoc.*, 78, 15, 1953.

86. **Baker, R. A., Hillman, B. J., McLennnan, J. E., Strand, R. D., and Kaufman, S. M.,** Sequelae of Metrizamide myelography in 200 examinations, *Am. J. Roentgenol.*, 130, 499, 1978.

87. **Ahlgren, P.,** Amipaque myelographie. The side effects compared with Dimer X, *Neuroradiology*, 9, 197, 1975.

88. **Hindmarsh, T., Grepe, A., and Widen, L.,** Metrizamide-phenothiazine interaction, *Acta Radiol. Diagn.*, 16, 129, 1975.

89. **Skalpe, I. O.,** The toxicity of the non-ionic water-soluble contrast medium Metrizamide (Amipaque) in selective vertebral angiography, *Neuroradiology*, 13, 19, 1977.

90. **Kaada, B.,** Transient EEG abnormalities following lumbar myelography with Metrizamide, *Acta Radiol. Diagn.*, Suppl. 335, 380, 1973.

91. **Lundervold, A. and Sortland, O.,** EEG disturbances following myelography, cisternography, and ventriculography with Metrizamide, *Acta Radiol Diagn.*, Suppl. 355, 379, 1977.

92. **Tourtellotte, W. W., Henderson, W. G., Tucker, R. P., Gilland, O., Walker, J. E., and Kokman, E.,** A randomised, double-blind clinical trial comparing the 22 versus 26 gauge needle in the production of the post-lumbar puncture syndrome in normal individuals, *Headache*, 12, 73, 1972.

93. **Irstam, L. and Sellden, U.,** Adverse effects of lumbar myelography with Amipaque and Dimer X, *Acta Radiol Diagn.*, 17, 145, 1976.

94. **Grainger, R. G., Kendall, B. E., Wylie, I. G.,** Lumbar myelography with Metrizamide: a non-ionic contrast medium, *Br. J. Radiol.*, 49, 996, 1976.

95. **Tourtellotte, W. W., Haerer, A. F., Heller, G. L., and Somers, J. E.,** *Post-Lumbar Puncture Headache*, Charles C Thomas, Springfield, Ill., 1964.

96. **Skalpe, I. O.,** Adverse effects of water-soluble contrast media in myelography, cisternography and ventriculography. A review with special reference to Metrizamide, *Acta Radiol. Diagn.*, Suppl. 355, 359, 1977.

97. **Potts, D. G., Gomez, D. G., and Abbott, G. F.,** Possible causes of complications of myelography with water-soluble contrast medium, *Acta Radiol. Diagn.*, Suppl. 355, 390, 1977.

98. **Hilal, S. K., Dauth, G. W., Burger, L. C., and Gilman, S.,** Effect of isotonic contrast agents on spinal reflexes in the cat, *Radiology*, 122, 149, 1977.

99. **Gonsette, R. E.,** Advances in ventriculography and myelography with the nonionic contrast medium Metrizamide, *Acta Radiol. Diagn.*, Suppl. 347, 467, 1975.

100. **Buruma, O. J. and Hekster, R. E. M.,** Transient areflexia following thoracolumbar myelography with Metrizamide. Report of a case, *Acta Radiol. Diagn.*, Suppl. 355, 371, 1977.

101. **Amundsen, P.,** Metrizamide in cervical myelography. Survey and present state, *Acta Radiol. Diagn.*, Suppl. 355, 403, 1977.

102. **Sortland, O., Lundervold, A., and Nesbakken, R.,** Mental confusion and epileptic seizures following cervical myelography with Metrizamide. Report of a case, *Acta Radiol. Diagn.*, Suppl. 355, 403, 1977.

103. **Berg Hansen, E., Fahrenkrug, A., and Praestholm, J.,** Late meningeal effects of myelographic contrast media with special reference to Metrizamide, *Br. J. Radiol.*, 51, 321, 1978.

104. **Ahlgren, P.,** Amipaque myelography without late adhesive arachnoidal changes, *Neuroradiology*, 14, 231, 1978.

105. **Wylie, I. G., Afshar, F., and Koeze, T. H.,** Results of the use of a new water-soluble contrast medium (Metrizamide) in the posterior fossa of the baboon, *Br. J. Radiol.*, 18, 1007, 1975.

106. **Halaburt, H. and Lester, J.,** Leptomeningeal changes following lumbar myelography with water-soluble contrast media (meglumine iothalamate and methiodal sodium), *Neuroradiology*, 5, 70, 1973.

107. **Skalpe, I. O.,** Adhesive arachnoiditis following lumbar radiculography with water-soluble contrast agents, *Radiology*, 121, 647, 1976.

108. **Haughton, V. M., Ho, K. C., and Unger, F. G.,** Arachnoiditis following myelography with water-soluble agents, *Radiology*, 125, 731, 1977.

109. **Raedberg, C. and Wennberg, E.,** Late sequelae following lumbar myelography with water-soluble contrast media, *Acta Radiol. Diagn.*, 14, 507, 1973.

110. **Haughton, V. M., Ho, K. C., Larson, S. J., Unger, G. F., and Correa-Paz, F.,** Experimental production of arachnoiditis with water-soluble myelographic media, *Radiology*, 123, 681, 1977.

111. **Haughton, V. M., Ho, K. C., Unger, G. F., Larson, S. J., Williams, A. L., and Eldevik, A. P.,** Severity of postmyelographic arachnoiditis and concentration of meglumine iocarmate in primates, *Am. J. Roentgenol.*, 130, 313, 1978.

112. **Irstam, L. and Rosencrantz, M.,** Water soluble contrast media and adhesive arachnoiditis. I. Reinvestigation of nonoperated cases, *Acta Radiol. Diagn.*, 14, 497, 1973.

113. **Irstam, L. and Rosencrantz, M.,** Water-soluble contrast media and adhesive arachnoiditis. II. Reinvestigation of operated cases, *Acta Radiol. Diagn.*, 15, 1, 1974.

114. **Yuen, T. G. H., Agnew, W. F., and Rumbough, C. L.,** Ultrastructural effects of Conray 60 and Pantopaque on ependyma and choroid plexus following intraventricular injection, *Invest. Radiol.,* 11, 112, 1976.
115. **Piwonka, R. W., Healey, J. E., and Rosenberg, F. J.,** Intrathecal tolerance of Metrizamide in choralose anesthetized cats, *Invest. Radiol.,* 11, 182, 1976.
116. **Cecil, J. P., Regnier, G., Guaquiere, A., Deffiny, L., and Cuevelier, A.,** Postural protection against complications in radiculography with Dimer X, *Neuroradiology,* 7, 167, 1974.
117. **Berner, A. and Johansen, J. G.,** Histologic effects of Amipaque (Metrizamide) and various contrast media on mouse peritoneum, *Invest. Radiol.,* 13, 161, 1978.

Chapter 7

NORMAL MYELOGRAM

A normal myelogram is commonly divided into lumbosacral, thoracic, and cervical sections. This radiologic, topographic division does not correspond to the anatomic and clinical segments of the spinal cord but rather to the type of examination and the anatomic area presented on myelograms. A normal myelogram is in essence a fluoroscopic and radiographic presentation of the subarachnoid space filled with either positive or negative contrast media. The subarachnoid space being a three dimensional cavity requires multiple radiographic projections to reach an estimate of its diameters, size, and shape.

In the frontal projection of the lumbosacral area, the width of the column of the radiopaque contrast medium in the subarachnoid space varies from approximately 15 to 25 mm. The opaque column narrows in the caudad direction, usually ending at the level of S_1 in a conic fashion (Figure 1).* The shape and length of the sacral end of the subarachnoid space can also vary.[1] The volume of the subarachnoid space in the lumbar region can be estimated by the amount of contrast medium necessary to fill it to the level of the third lumbar vertebral body. If the space is within the normal limits, approximately 8 to 12 cc are required, and if it is narrow, about 6 cc of the contrast agent will be sufficient. The narrowness of the subarachnoid space may sometimes owe its appearance to a congenitally narrow spinal canal or wide epidural space.[2] The size of the subarachnoid space can equally change under physiological conditions associated with coughing, sneezing, or other kinds of straining.

The column of the contrast medium in the anteroposterior projection of the lumbar area has a symmetrical appearance. On its both sides, convex extensions of the arachnoid sleeves are seen surrounding the exiting nerves (Figure 2). If the patient is rotated into an accentuated anterior oblique position, the arachnoid pouches are well projected (Figure 3). Radiolucent lines representing the nerves can be visualized within the arachnoid sleeves when the contrast medium fills the space between the nerve roots and the lateral surface of the subarachnoid space (Figure 4). The subarachnoid space surrounding the nerve roots varies in size, and occasionally it appears wider and longer showing on myelograms a cyst-like dilatation (Figure 5). The arachnoid sleeves and the nerves are turned downwards and laterally, and they can be seen more clearly if the patient remains for a shorter period of time in the erect posture.[3-6]

Lateral radiographs in a semierect position of the patient will delineate the anterior surface of the opaque column of the contrast medium (Figure 2). This view can provide information on the relationship between the ventral portion of the subarachnoid space and the epidural space and bony structures. The anterior margin of the subarachnoid space can have either a smooth, convex, or flat appearance. If a smaller quantity of the insoluble contrast agent is used, the anterior margin of the opaque column can be interrupted in the prone position of the patient, and the contrast medium will tend to pool between intervertebral spaces thus forming an "hour-glass" configuration. If a larger amount of the opaque medium is added, this hour-glass appearance of the anterior surface of the opaque column will change. The nerve roots and arachnoid sleeves can be outlined in the upper lumbar area on radiographs using a horizontal beam with the patient in the right or left lateral decubitus. The thickness of the epidural space

* All figures appear following the text.

varies, and it appears on lateral or oblique projections as a radiolucent zone between the column of the opaque contrast medium and the bony structures (Figure 2). Usually, the epidural space is wider in the lumbosacral region and becomes narrower in the upper levels of the lumbar spine (Figure 2). The size of the epidural space depends also upon the position of the patient. In the upright position, the epidural space has the tendency to become narrower because the spinal venous plexus contains relatively less blood than when the patient is prone. These changes in the size of the epidural space will cause alterations in the shape of the opaque column. If the width of the epidural space is especially pronounced, the column of the opaque contrast medium can be reduced in size considerably. On the other hand, if the epidural space is narrow, the column of the contrast medium will appear much wider and almost adjacent to the bony structures.

When dynamic studies of the lumbosacral area are carried out, the patient's normal myelographic anatomy changes depending upon his position. In extension, the anterior margin of the opaque column appears to be much closer to the posterior surface of the vertebral bodies, and behind the intervertebral spaces indentations on the radiopaque column may appear. In anterior flexion of the spine, the ventral surface of the subarachnoid space is detached from intervertebral spaces and the prominence of disks is less evident. The length of the conus of the subarachnoid space varies between the upper border of S_1 to S_3 (see Chapter 4, Figures 1, 4, and 5). This anatomic variation can be, at times, the cause of some diagnostic problems because if the sacral end of the subarachnoid space is short, pathologic processes involving the lower epidural space cannot be visualized. It should be mentioned that the sacral end of the subarachnoid space narrows gradually, not only in its transverse but also in its ventrodorsal diameter and it is more separated from the bony structures of the spinal canal.

The nerve filaments of the cauda equina can be well visualized when water-soluble contrast media are used. With insoluble opaque media, they can be, to some extent, demonstrated on radiographs with the patient in the semierect posture applying a more penetrating beam. (See Chapter 4, Figure 1.) The nerves appear as linear radiolucencies, mostly divergent on frontal projection, and as diagonal radiolucent lines directed downward and ventrally in the lateral view. With insoluble contrast media, it is difficult to estimate whether the nerves are normal or not unless a considerable edema is present (Figure 2). With water-soluble contrast media, however, this evaluation is considerably simplified.

The upper lumbar and lower thoracic regions of the subarachnoid space are explored with the patient in an approximately horizontal position (Figure 6). Using insoluble opaque media, the conus of the spinal cord is visualized occasionally as a radiolucency at the level of T_{12} to L_1. The anterior spinal artery can form a slender radiolucent line in the region of the conus. The demonstration of the anterior spinal artery can approximately demarcate the location of the conus. If it is necessary to determine more precisely the size and shape of the lower segment of the spinal cord, the needle should be withdrawn and the patient turned on his back. With the utilization of Metrizamide®, the visualization of the conus is achieved in a much more reliable way.

The thoracic subarachnoid space opacified by the opaque medium is about 15 mm wide in the frontal projection. Here, it appears wider in the region of the lumbar enlargement of the spinal cord and can exceed 22 mm in width at the T_{11} to T_{12} level. Above the lumbar enlargement of the spinal cord, the opaque column becomes gradually narrower reaching its minimal transverse diameter at about T_9 level. The second enlargement of the spinal cord widens the column at about T_1 level. Symmetrical convex pouchings of the column may be sometimes seen at the level of each vertebral pedicle, representing the opaque medium in the arachnoid sleeves around the nerves.

Often, these arachnoid pouchings are not demonstrated because of incomplete filling. The column of the insoluble opaque medium in the thoracic area is thin and cannot always reach the arachnoid sleeves (see Chapter 2, Figure 2; Chapter 4, Figure 6). Radiographs in the lateral decubitus with a horizontal beam will outline more adequately the subarachnoid space around the nerve roots. The dorsal spinal cord appears in the frontal projection as a radiolucent band situated in the middle portion of the vertebral canal encompassed by the contrast medium in the subarachnoid gutters. Occasionally, a thin, linear radiolucency representing the anterior spinal artery divides the cord almost into two halves in the longitudinal direction.[4] Its radicular contributors can be seen following the nerves and joining the main trunk of the anterior spinal artery (Figure 6).

The cross-table lateral projection in the patient's prone position demonstrates a smooth or angulated concave margin of the column of the contrast medium (Figure 6). The ventral epidural space in the thoracic area is usually quite thin (Figure 6). Normal protrusions of the intervertebral spaces can be quite prominent. Characteristically, the irregularities of the opaque column observed in the thoracic area are often inconstant and occasionally cannot be recognized if the passage of the contrast medium is repeated. Cineradiography is often helpful in the evaluation of the anatomic myelographic features of the thoracic subarachnoid space. Metrizamide® and radiolucent contrast agents will provide more information about the thoracic area than radiopaque insoluble contrast media (Figure 7).

In oblique or lateral views, the dentate ligament may be seen separating the anterior from the posterior thoracic subarachnoid compartment. The pulsatile movements of the contrast medium are not pronounced in the midthoracic area, but they become apparent in its caudad and cephalad regions.

In the frontal projection, the cervical area in its distal part shows an enlargement representing cervical intumescence. The width of the intumescence is maximal at the level of C_5 to C_6 and it gradually diminishes downward to the level of T_2 and upwards to C_3. The subarachnoid space appears wide and measures approximately 30 mm. The spinal cord is visualized situated in the middle of the subarachnoid space occupying about two thirds of its width (see Chapter 2, Figure 2; this chapter, Figure 6). With an adequate exposure, the cervical spinal cord can be well outlined on positive contrast myelograms (Pantopaque® or Metrizamide®) and its transverse diameter is accessible to measurements. However, measurements of the sagittal diameter of the spinal cord are difficult to determine with insoluble contrast media; therefore, gas myelography would still be the procedure of choice to establish its values (see Chapter 2, Figures 7 and 9). The values of the transverse and sagittal diameters of the spinal cord were discussed in Chapter 2.

In the cervical region, the nerve roots are usually well outlined surrounded by arachnoid outpouchings that can be quite wide and occasionally triangular in shape (Figures 6 and 8). The nerves are seen passing obliquely in the caudal direction forming the apex of the encircling arachnoid space (Figure 9). The nerves appear symmetrical on both sides of the subarachnoid space. They have an almost horizontal position in the upper cervical area and become more diagonal in the lower cervical and upper thoracic regions. It is possible to distinguish the lower cervical nerve roots that form the brachial plexus as thicker and more prominent linear radiolucencies. The lower cervical nerves are seen to originate from the spinal cord at a higher level than their exit through intervertebral foramina (Figure 6). The posterior root, when demonstrated on radiographs in supine position, appears to be larger than the anterior. If the contrast medium is accumulated in the lateral subarachnoid gutters, the anterior spinal artery will be visualized as an almost vertical radiolucent line dividing the cord into two halves.

(See Chapter 2, Figure 8; this chapter, Figure 6.) In the cervical region, the radicular arteries can be well discerned on myelograms as they converge towards the anterior spinal artery. It is usually possible to differentiate the rootlets from the radiolucency of the radicular arteries. The arteries are further seen reaching the anterior spinal artery, and the rootlets extending to the spinal cord. In oblique positions with adequate filling of the subarachnoid gutters, the dentate ligament can be recognized as a thin, linear radiolucency directed vertically between the dorsal nerve roots and the homogenous opacity of the contrast medium in the ventral compartment (Figures 6 and 9). The ligament is ordinarily thicker in the cervical area; it can be demonstrated readily and its visualization may prove helpful for the determination of the position of the cervical spinal cord. In the upper region of the cervical subarachnoid space, the contrast medium separates into two columns surrounding an eliptic radiolucency that represents the dens epistrophei (Figure 6). By gently rotating the patient's head the cranial end of the opaque column will diverge and flow around the dens. The two bands of the contrast medium surrounding the dens will then merge at its cranial end forming a homogenous radiopacity extending forward in the direction of the clivus. If the head is flexed, the area of the clivus will be clearly outlined; on the other hand, if the head is extended, the contrast medium will flow into the opposite direction, that is, into the cisterna magna. The cisterna magna will be also filled if the head and neck are turned into oblique or lateral positions. The directed movements of the head and neck are important for the demonstration of the normal anatomy of the upper cervical area.[5]

The filling of the upper cervical region wtih Metrizamide® can outline very well the anatomical structures involved. The lesser density of Metrizmide® provides a more distinguishable appearance of the elements seen in myelographic anatomy. Furthermore, the coating of the pia with this contrast agent can be achieved more successfully than with insoluble contrast agents.

With the patient prone, the cross-table lateral radiographs present the ventral compartment of the subarachnoid space and the anterior margin of the spinal cord (see Volume 2, Chapter 2, Figure 1). The spinal cord is detached from the ventral surface of the arachnoid space approximately 3 to 4 mm. If the opaque contrast medium fills the anterior and posterior compartments, the dorsal surface of the spinal cord will be outlined (see Volume 2, Chapter 2, Figure 1). The distance between the margin of the spinal cord and the ventral surface of the subarachnoid space depends, to some extent, on the position of the patient's head. In hyperextension, the width of the contrast medium can be 5 mm or more. The column of the opaque medium outlined tangentially in the lateral view has a smooth, convex, or slightly undulated curve (see Chapter 10, Figure 14). If the films are sufficiently exposed using a higher kV technique, the anterior margin of the cord can be seen as well as the linear curve of the dentate ligament. The ventral aspect of the spinal cord may be more radiolucent, assumably because of the presence of the anterior rootlets and pial vessels (see Volume 2, Chapter 2, Figure 1). In the upper cervical area, the opaque column of the contrast medium appears displaced posteriorly due to the presence of the dens and the transverse ligament, the width of which can vary considerably (see Chapter 4, Figure 10). The anterior margin of the column of the contrast medium will form a concave curve over this region which is mostly smooth. If the dens is less prominent and the thickness of the ligaments not increased, the Pantopaque® column may have a more horizontal appearance. As the column flows over the dens, it gradually moves into the subarachnoid space on the dorsal surface of the clivus (see Chapter 4, Figure 10). In the lateral projection, the dorsal margin of the cervical subarachnoid space appears either with a convex or horizontal border, and is influenced by the thickness of the ligamentum flavum.

The contrast medium, as it fills the dorsal region of the clivus, will outline the vertebral arteries, their junction, and the basilar artery in the frontal projection (Figure 10). The branches of these arteries can be also demonstrated, especially the inferior posterior cerebellar arteries. The origin of the hypoglossal nerve can be seen under the margin of the foramen magnum. In oblique positions, it is possible to outline the cisterna magna, the cerebellar tonsillae, the cerebello-pontine cistern, the trigeminal nerve, and, if necessary, the auditory canal. The number of anatomic details that can be shown in the upper cervical area and in the region of the base of the skull depends to some extent upon the experience of the investigator and the applied technique.[1-3,5,6]

In the course of the exploration of the cervico-occipital junction, the vigorous pulsations in the cervical area as well as the straining of the patient can cause a sudden flow of the contrast medium into the cranial direction. Coughing can be useful if the patient is in the erect position so that small droplets of the contrast medium can be collected from the base of the skull and the upper cervical region.

At times, it is necessary to turn the patient in the supine position to explore the posterior subarachnoid compartment, posterior aspects of the foramen magnum, and the cisterna magna (see Chapter 8, Figure 2). In the supine posture, the opaque contrast medium has the tendency to aggragate in the lateral gutters and form a frame around the spinal cord that appears in the anteroposterior projection as a radiolucent band (see Chapter 9, Figure 5). In the cross-table lateral view, the cisterna magna and the dorsal compartment of the subarachnoid space will be well filled with the contrast medium. The width of the dorsal subarachnoid space is narrower than that of the ventral compartment. In the supine position, the dorsal nerve roots, and occasionally posterior spinal arteries, the septum posticum, and the posterior nerve rootlets can be visualized.

I. TECHNICALLY INADEQUATE MYELOGRAM

A faulty myelographic procedure can be attributed to the lumbar puncture, instillation of the contrast medium, radiographic technique, or individual inexperience, and it can cause diagnostic errors. A common source of difficulty is the diagnostic lumbar puncture preceding myelography within a short period of time. It can produce a leakage of the CSF into the subdural or epidural spaces. The accumulation of the spinal fluid that leaked into the subdural space will separate the dura from the arachnoid and form a pool (subdural hydroma) compressing the subarachnoid space. In this way, the needle inserted for myelography can be located in the subdural space and the return flow of the spinal fluid may be quite profuse. The instillation of the contrast medium under these circumstances will occur into the subdural space. If the diagnostic lumbar puncture is performed, we prefer for the above reasons to delay the myelographic procedure for 1 week to 10 days, or to perform a suboccipital puncture. Multiple traumatic punctures linked to myelography can produce the same effect. Therefore, the puncture should be performed precisely and the subarachnoid space perforated by the needle at one location only. If the bevel of the needle or the tip of the stylet are not sharp, they can displace the arachnoid anteriorly and the needle will be only partially inserted in the subarachnoid space. Equally, if the needle is not sufficiently inserted into the subarachnoid space, one segment of the bevel can remain in the subdural fissure. In both instances, the contrast medium will be injected into the subdural space. It is also possible to inject the contrast medium into the anterior subdural space if the needle perforates the ventral arachnoid wall. These defects induced by the puncture can cause diagnostic errors resulting from the narrowing of the subarachnoid space.[2]

Subdural instillation of the contrast medium is a common technical deficiency. If a water-soluble contrast medium is injected into the subdural space, it might be difficult to recognize promptly its location since its spreading is rather fast. The insoluble contrast medium, if injected into the subdural space, will move slowly, and the pulsatile movements and the free flow characteristic of the subarachnoid instillation will be absent. If the patient is asked to cough or strain, the movement of the contrast agent will be barely apparent. A cross-table lateral radiograph in this situation may prove helpful because it will demonstrate the position of the needle and the presence of a larger amount of Pantopaque® in the subdural space. If the table is tilted head down, the contrast medium will move slowly in the cranial direction, in an irregular fashion often broken into several longer or shorter linear layers that follow the main column. Characteristically, the usual shape of the sacral end of the subarachnoid space cannot be demonstrated. Equally, the pooling of the contrast medium in the subarachnoid space due to gravity cannot be seen on the cross-table lateral views. It is known to be difficult to remove completely the insoluble contrast medium injected into the subdural space.[1-3]

The installation of the contrast medium into the epidural space is less frequent and it can occur if a larger collection of the CSF is present in the epidural tissue as a result of a puncture performed prior to myelography. The diffuse, rapid flow of the contrast medium in the soft epidural tissue is quite typical and can be recognized promptly on fluoroscopy. If this happens, the injection of the contrast medium should stop immediately. The contrast medium can escape thorough the intervertebral foramina following the spinal nerves and can be distinguished in the soft tissues surrounding the spine.

The penetration of the contrast medium into the ventricles or intracranial cisterns should be prevented because the meningeal reaction with an increase of body temperature can complicate the myelographic procedure (see Chapter 6, Figures 1 and 3). In addition, other complications may occur, as was mentioned in the text concerning this matter.

A faulty radiographic technique producing over- or underexposed films can further on be the source of diagnostic errors. Such errors should be avoided because the patient is exposed to considerable radiation in the course of myelography.[7] The myelographic technique should be planned in such a way that the patient is exposed to the least possible radiation dose, in particular if a child is the subject of examination.

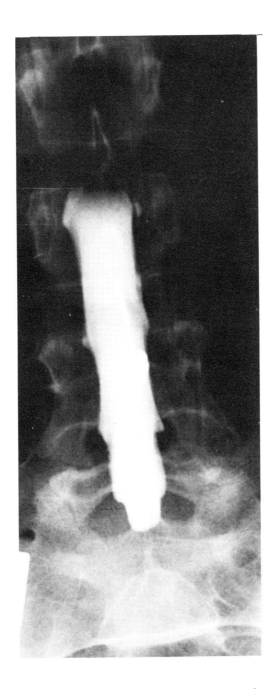

FIGURE 1. Lumbar myelogram in anteroposterior view demarcates the subarachnoid sac with obliquely positioned nerve roots. The sac end at S_1 has a rounded appearance.

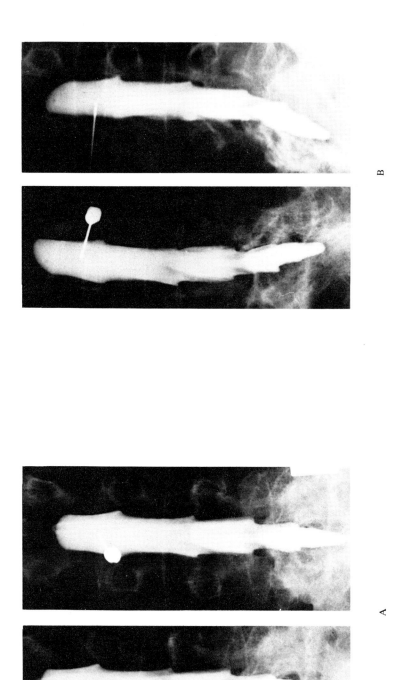

A

B

FIGURE 2 (A).   Normal lumbar Pantopaque® myelogram in the prone anteroposterior position demonstrates clearly the nerve roots and the surrounding meningeal sheaths. At the level of L_5 to S_1 the subarachnoid space is slightly narrowed. (B) The lumbar nerve roots and meningeal sleeves on myelograms in the oblique upright position. (C) The presentation of the lower and upper segments of the lumbar area. At Th_{12} the radiolucency of the lumbar enlargement of the spinal cord is noticeable. (D) Lateral projection shows the arachnoid sac well filled with the contrast. The position of the needle can be evaluated on all myelograms. At L_5 to S_1 level, the subarachnoid space is compressed by the ligament and minimal spondylolisthesis.

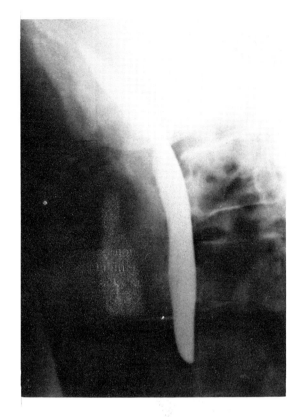

FIGURE 2D

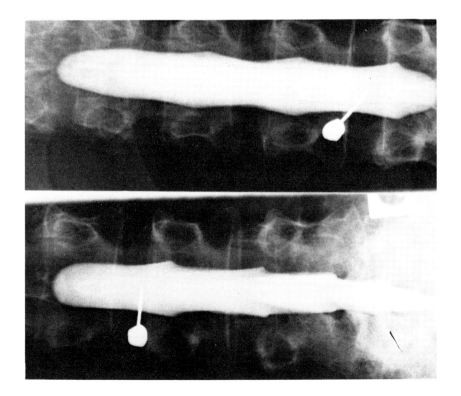

FIGURE 2C

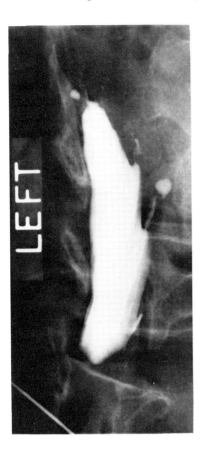
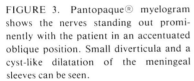

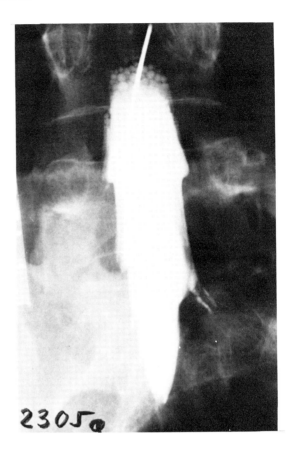

FIGURE 3. Pantopaque® myelogram shows the nerves standing out prominently with the patient in an accentuated oblique position. Small diverticula and a cyst-like dilatation of the meningeal sleeves can be seen.

FIGURE 4. Lumbar Pantopaque® myelogram in a slightly oblique position of the patient outlines the nerves. Far out on the arachnoid sac a nerve can be visualized encompassed by the contrast medium in the meningeal sleeves.

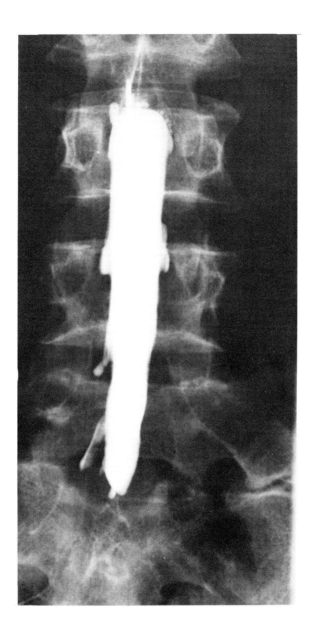

FIGURE 5. The meningeal sleeves accompanying the nerves appear long; some of the sleeves form small diverticula or cyst-like formations. The patient was rotated minimally, to demonstrate clearly the exiting lumbar nerves.

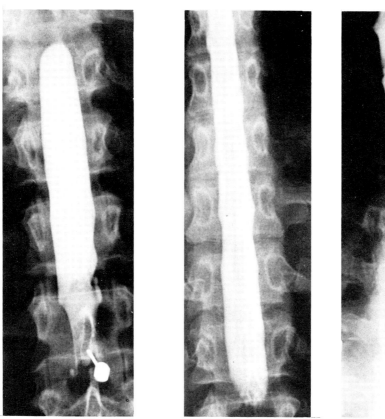
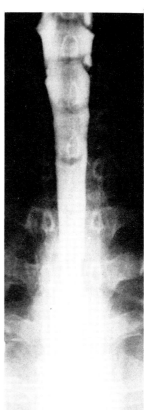

A   B   C

FIGURE 6(A).   The flow of Pantopaque® in the upper lumbar and lower thoracic areas is seen in the form of a solid radiopaque column. (B) The thoracic area is filled with opaque contrast medium, and the spinal cord with its nerve roots is apparent because the contrast was distributed thinly. Both the lumbar enlargement of the spinal cord and the anterior spinal artery are visualized; however, the latter is much better delineated. The meningeal sleeves appear flat. (C) Pantopaque® fills the thoracic and lower cervical areas and the column of the contrast becomes narrower in the thoracic region as it flows cranially. (D) Oblique view of the cervical area. The nerve roots and meningeal sleeves are clearly marked, whereas the margin of the spinal cord can be just recognized. The exits of the nerve roots are more horizontal than in the thoracic or lumbar region. (E) The opposite oblique projection reveals the nerve roots, some tributary arteries reaching the anterior spinal artery, and a small bony spur at C_5 compressing a meningeal sleeve. (F) Cervical Pantopaque® myelogram in the prone anteroposterior projection exhibits the spinal cord encompassed by the subarachnoid gutters filled with the contrast medium. The nerve roots can be seen all the way from the spinal cord to their exits, having an almost horizontal position. Also, the anterior spinal artery and some of its tributaries are demonstrated. (G) The contrast medium fills the lower and upper cervical area, and the spinal cord with the nerve roots is well outlined. (H) Here, the contrast flows around the dens that appears as an eliptic radiolucent structure. The cranial segment of the spinal cord is equally well delineated, the spinal artery apparent, as well as the tributary arteries joining the main arterial trunk. (I) "Swimmer's" view of the cervicothoracic junction.

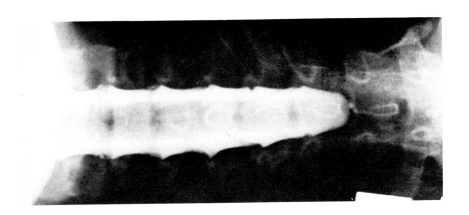

FIGURE 6F

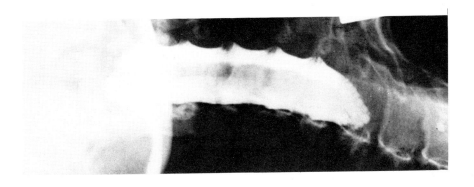

FIGURE 6E

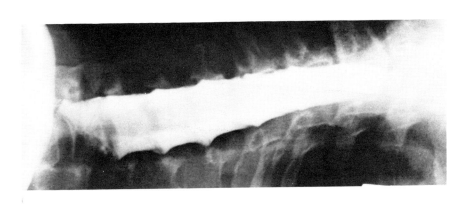

FIGURE 6D

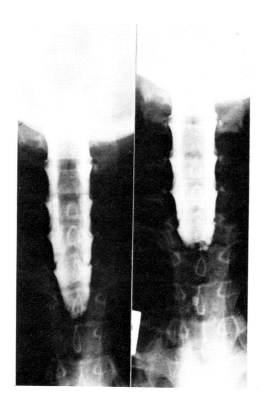

FIGURE 6G

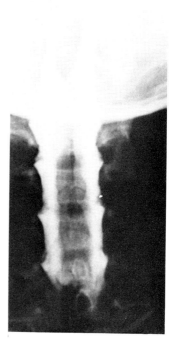

FIGURE 6H

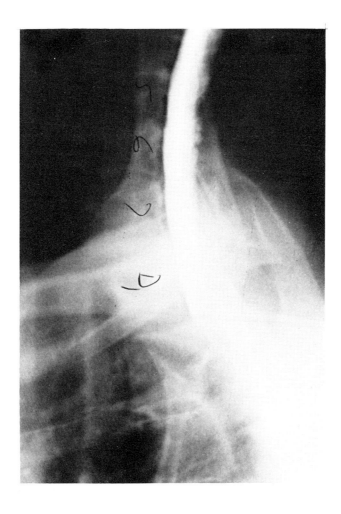

FIGURE 61

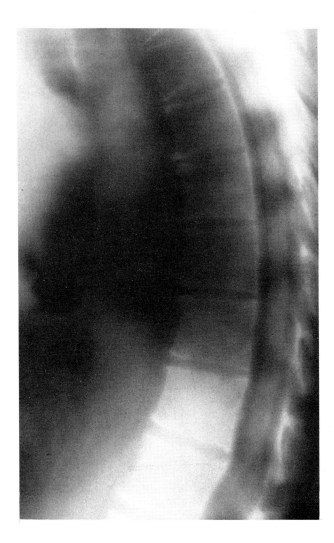

FIGURE 7.   Gas myelogram of the thoracic region demarcates the spinal cord and the subarachnoid space from the bony structure of the spinal canal. The ventral epidural space is seen as a thin radiolucent line along the dorsal surface of the vertebrae.

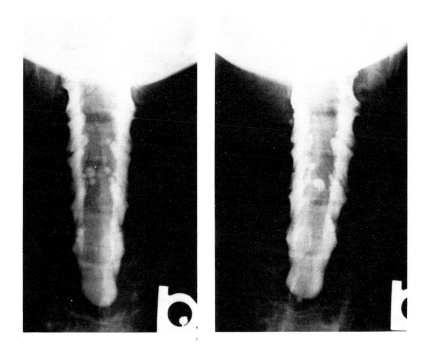

FIGURE 8. Myelogram of the proximal cervical region, anteroposterior view. The spinal cord is seen well demarcated with the nerve roots. Globulation of Pantopaque® covers some areas of the spinal cord.

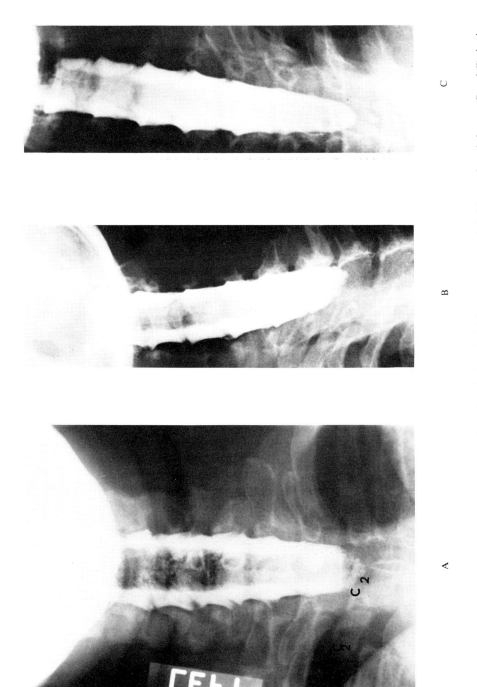

FIGURE 9(A).   Prone, anteroposterior myelogram outlines the spinal cord with its nerve roots encircled by meningeal sleeves. (B and C)   In the oblique position, the exiting nerve roots can be seen as well as the entering tributary arteries.

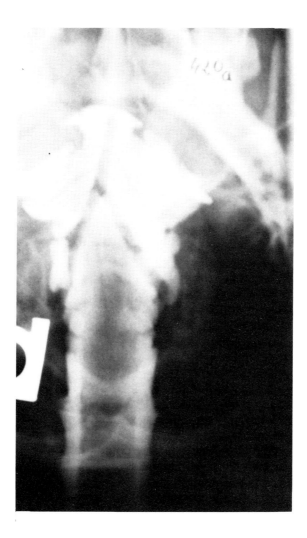

FIGURE 10. Normal anatomy of the cervico-cranial junction. The vertebral and basilar arteries are seen with their emerging branches. The origin of the anterior spinal artery is recognizable.

REFERENCES

1. Shapiro, R., *Myelography,* 3rd ed., Year Book Medical Publishers, Chicago, 1975, chap. 7.
2. Taveras, J. M. and Wood, E. H., *Diagnostic Neuroradiology,* Vol. 2 (Part 7), Williams & Wilkins, Baltimore, 1976.
3. Epstein, B. S., *The Spine,* 4th ed., Lea & Febiger, Philadelphia, 1976, chap. 5.
4. Ranson, S. W. and Clark, S. L., *The Anatomy of the Nervous System,* 10th ed., W. B. Saunders Philadelphia, 1966, chap. 2.
5. Deckers, K., *Klinische Neuroradiologie,* Georg Thieme Verlag, Stuttgart, 1960, 79.
6. Rothman, R. H. and Simeone, F. A., *The Spine,* W. B. Saunders, Philadelphia, 1975.
7. Rohrer, R. H., Sprawls, P., Jr., Miller, W. B., Jr., and Weens, H. S., Radiation doses received in myelographic examinations, *Radiology,* 82, 106, 1964.

Chapter 8

MYELOGRAPHY IN DEVELOPMENTAL MALFORMATIONS

The main differentiation of the components of the central nervous system (CNS) is laid down about the 8th week of fetal life. In that period, various noxious agents can affect the fetus and cause a complete absence (aplasia, agenesis), partial absence (hypoplasia), or changes in structure and organization (dysplasia) of different segments of the CNS. Up to approximately six months of embryonic development, already formed components of the CNS, including the spinal cord, can be affected by noxious agents and resorbed with little inflammatory or glial reaction. Hence, it may be difficult to differentiate the alterations of the spinal cord that occur due to the destruction of the formed nervous tissue from those produced by arrested development. A lesion present at birth does not necessarily imply that its origin is hereditary. Actually, most congenital malformations are not inherited. In most instances, it is difficult to identify the injurious agent responsible for the fetal lesion. Malnutrition, vitamin deficiencies, anoxia, exposure to endogenous or exogenous toxins or infections, hypoglycemia, ionizing radiation, are some of the factors that can cause the occurrence of congenital anomalies of the nervous system.[18]

The classifications of congenital malformations of the spinal cord are morphologic, etiologic, or clinical. The morphologic classification is more applicable to the radiologic exploration of the spinal cord because it indicates anatomic relationships, functional connections, and developmental sequences. Some of these developmental malformations concerning the spinal cord and meninges, which can be recognized by radiologic techniques, will be the topic of this text.

I. DIASTEMATOMYELIA

Diastematomyelia (diastomyelia, diplomyelia) represents a division of the spinal cord into two longitudinal entities, each surrounded with its own meningeal fold. The spinal canal in this malformation may be abnormally wide or even duplicated, and spina bifida is usually present (Figure 1)*. The arachnoid and the dura are duplicated in approximately half the cases, but the pia is always.[4,5,18] A spicule of bone, or band of cartilage, or fibrocartilaginous tissue separates the spinal cord into two halves, attached commonly anteriorly to the body of one or more vertebrae and dorsally to the neural arch. Thus split cord is fixed by this spicule or a fibrous band, and in the course of the growth of the spinal canal, the traction of the cord evolves. The division of the cord may involve one or more segments, but not all the levels of the spinal cord. Diastematomyelia is often associated with malformations of the vertebrae, changes of the skin, Anrold-Chiari malformation, syringomyelia, or meningomyelocele.[6-8]

Explanations of the etiology of disastematomyelia presented in literature are manifold. It is believed that the malformation takes place primarily in the spinal cord and that the changes in the bones and skin are secondary.[9] It is postulated that the lower segments of the cord develop from a solid bundle of cells instead of a tube, and that two cavities are formed within the cord failing to fuse into a single central canal in the normal way.[1] Another theory suggests that the infolding of the walls of the neural

---

* All figures appear following the text.

tube omitting to fuse with the neural plate is the cause of this malformation.[2] In some instances, persistent neurenteric canal divides the spinal cord into two halves. Some investigators consider that this arrangement is common in diastematomyelia, and that the spur seen in this condition is formed out of neurenteric canal.[3-9]

Diastematomyelia is more common in females and children, but it can be seen in adult men as well.[4,8] The usual site of this malformation is the thoracolumbar area, but it was also found in the cervical, upper dorsal, and lumbar regions. Accompanying clinical signs are connected to the fixation and splitting of the spinal cord, and to the associated anomalies such as thickening of the skin, pigmentation covered by hair, a sinus tract, or a dimple, all of which can be seen at the level of diastematomyelia. Further on, lipoma, meningocele, various abnormalities of the bony spinal canal can also cause a midline lump.[7,10,11] With the growth of the spinal canal the atrophy of one of the lower limbs may appear, as well as enuresis, absence of knee and ankle jerks, loss of cutaneous sensation and extensor plantar responses, paraplegic disorders, changes in gait, different deformities of feet and eventually trophic ulcerations.[5-7,11] The severity of these clinical manifestations will depend upon the extent of the division of the spinal cord and its fixation. An incomplete division may be asymtomatic. In extreme cases of complete doubling of a longer segment of the cord, various clinical signs will be pronounced. The stretching of the cord can ensue from the presence of the bony spurs, but also from the fibrous bands connecting the spinal cord to the subcutaneous tissues associated with defects in the neural arches, dermoids, neurofibromas, and intraspinal lipomas. The cause of the cord fixation should be identified because its removal is necessary most of the time.[5-7,11]

The radiologic findings of diastematomyelia consist of the demonstration of the bony spur, widening of the spinal canal, and multiple anomalies of the bony spinal canal (Figure 1). The visualization of the spicule depends upon its ossification. It can be seen as a 1- to 2-cm long bony partition directed often from below upwards, usually of an elliptic shape. The bony spurs can be multiple, or absent if the fibrous or cartilagenous tissue bands divide the cord. The ossified spicule can be clearly demonstrated by means of tomography. Gas myelography outlines clearly the relationship of the bony spur to the spinal cord in the lateral and frontal views. Metrizamide® myelography should equally well demonstrate this defect. A myelogram, with opaque insoluble contrast media will show a midline filling defect that can have different shapes depending upon the size and contours of the spur. This defect can be seen in the prone position of the patient but, occasionally, the supine position might be more advantageous.[7,9,10] The caudal end of the conus, and the anterior spinal artery if seen on myelograms, can determine the extent of the spinal cord stretching. On myelograms, adhesions can be demonstrated as an additional feature.[7,10]

II. HYDROMYELIA

Hydromyelia should be distinguished from primary or secondary syringomyelia. The term hydromyelia derives from the dilatation of the central canal, the phenomenon that can be found in lesser degree in an otherwise normal spinal cord. There is a correlation between hydromyelia and developmental malformations of the neural tube. Hydromyelia can be associated with the spina bifida occulta, meningomyelocele, the Arnold-Chiari syndrome, and diastematomyelia. Usually, hydromyelia is not a progressive condition. It communicates with the central canal, and its walls are lined by ependymal cells. The central canal is dilated in a symmetrical way, and the cavity is situated centrally, mostly in the cervical area. There is no evidence of destruction of the adjacent tissue of the spinal cord. Occasionally, extensions of the cavity may simulate syringomyelia.[18,19]

Hydromyelia can cause a localized or more diffused enlargement of the spinal cord, which may be established on myelograms and often difficult to distinguish from syringomyelia or intramedullary expansive lesions. We applied gas myelography as the diagnostic procedure. According to some investigators who used Pantopaque® myelography, the penetration of the contrast medium into the dilated central canal could give a characteristic picture.[12] A more detailed description of the appearance of hydromyelia will be presented in the text concerning gas myelography.

III. THE ARNOLD-CHIARI MALFORMATION

The Arnold-Chiari malformation is considered to be a dysplasia of the cerebellum and the brain stem with caudal displacement of tongue-like extensions of the cerebellar hemispheres, amygdala, medulla, and the elongated fourth ventricle through the foramen magnum into the spinal canal. The downward cerebellar displacement was described by Arnold in 1894, in an infant, and later Chiari in 1895 completed the description of the malformation by adding his observations concerning the position of the cerebellar tonsillae and the medulla oblongata, and their relationship to the spinal cord in the cervical canal.[13,14] Chiari described three types of this malformation based on different variations linked to the descent of the components of the posterior fossa into the cervical canal. Numerous theories related to the development of this malformation have been advanced. For a longer period of time, the most attractive was the theory of fixation of the lower segment of the spinal cord and its inability to follow the growth of the spinal column. The origin of hydrocephalus, often associated with the Arnold-Chiari malformation, was explained by the stretching and narrowing of the aqueduct due to the caudal traction of the cerebellum. This thoery could not be fully sustained because it did not explain the absence of tension of the medulla and cervical cord and the relatively normal angulation of the thoracic and upper lumbar spinal nerves. In addition, experimental fixation of the spinal cord in the course of embryonic development in animals did not produce the Arnold-Chiari malformation.[15] A consideration was given to hydrocephalus as a possible etiological factor in the genesis of the Arnold-Chiari malformation. It was assumed that the herniation was caused by the pressure from above.[16,17] This, however, seems unlikely since the protruded cerebellar tissue represents dysplastic, redundant vermis, and amygdala.[18] Other researchers pointed out the role of hydromyelia in the genesis of the Arnold-Chiari malformation. Namely, it was supposed that the CSF leaked through the spinal canal into the amniotic sac, and that the increased intrauterine pressure on the fetal head forced the hindbrain into the spinal canal. It has been accepted by most investigators that the Arnold-Chiari malformation is a developmental malformation of the hindbrain, which probably occurs in the 3rd week of embryonic life.[17,18]

The pathologic findings show a tongue-like processus of dysplastic cerebellum extending downwards as far as C_3 or even C_7 behind the elongated medulla. The fourth ventrical is elongated and flattened. The foramina of Magendie an Luschka can extend below the foramen magnum and may be difficult to identify.[16,17] The Arnold-Chiari malformation presents itself in different forms. The displacement of the medulla and cerebellar vermis into the cervical canal can occur without involvement of the fourth ventricle. A mild or an arrested hydrocephalus can be linked to this asymptomatic form, often found in older children and adults representing Chiari's type I. In more severe cases, the lower part of the fourth ventricle and the medulla often overlap the upper cervical cord. The aqueduct is elongated, narrowed, and affected by gliosis that leads to internal hydrocephalus and the impairment of spinal fluid circulation. If the cerebellar tissue is impacted in the foramen magnum, a communicating hydrocephalus could be present. The lower part of the pons and the upper segment of the medulla show different changes in shape, usually thin and elongated, and the basilar artery deeply imbedded in the ventral surface of the pons.[18,19] A number of associated anomalies can complete the picture of the Arnold-Chiari malformation described as types II and III. There often is a lumbosacral myelomeningocele with fixation of the conus medullaris, and platypasia or basilar impression in which the atlas is fused with the skull. Furthermore, the posterior cranial fossa may be hypoplastic, the Klippel-Feil deformity can be present, too, and the existence of hydromyelia should not be excluded.[18-20] In the Arnold-Chiari malformation the lower cranial nerves are elongated, and the spinal nerves in the cervical area turned upwards in the direction of their exiting foramina.

Standard radiographs of the skull and cervical spine provide enough information about the anomalies of the bony structures. Nevertheless, myelography is an important diagnostic tool because not frequently will the clinical picture of the Arnold-Chiari malformation appear characteristic, but it will present itself as a disseminated sclerosis, or neoplasm of the cerebellum, brain stem, or the spinal cord. It can also simulate syringomyelia or arachnoiditis. Myelograms in the Arnold-Chiari malformation will demonstrate a lobulated symmetric filling defect created by herniated cerebellar tonsillae, or asymmetric if one tonsilla is lower than the other.[18,19] The filling defect on myelograms may be found as low as C_7. The myelographic examination in the supine position of the patient can provide more information in case opaque contrast media are used. In pronounced herniation of the tonsillae, the defect can be bilobulated, encompassed by narrow columns of the opaque medium extending towards the cisterna magna (Figure 2). Gas myelography can disclose cerebellar tonsillae as elongated densities, and frequently, the fourth ventricle can be identified below the foramen magnum. Gas can delineate the fourth ventricle and stenosis, or occlusion of the aqueduct. The demonstration of the cisterna magna by gas is often decisive. The establishing of the width of the cisterna may be of consequence not only for diagnostic but therapeutic purposes as well. Small filling defects pertaining to the tonsillae may be seen on gas myelography and missed on myelography with insoluble opaque contrast media. The myelographic features of the Arnold-Chiari malformation are not pathognomonic, for similar defects can be produced, for example, by a meningeoma at the cranio-spinal border. In meningeomas, the contour of the spinal cord is adjacent to the outlined tumor. In the Arnold-Chiari malformation, on the other hand, the displaced tonsillae usually do not show this demarcation between the two different tissues. An intramedullary tumor in the proximal cervical spinal cord leads through its generalized enlargement. If the position of the fourth ventricle is relatively unchanged, it will be even more difficult to differentiate an intramedullary tumor from the Arnold-Chiari malformation, or herniation of cerebellar tonsillae in an increased intracranial pressure.[12,18,19]

Sometimes, for differential diagnostic reasons, it is helpful to combine myelography with vertebral angiography. In the Arnold-Chiari syndrome, the displacement of the brain stem and the cerebellum through the foramen magnum into the upper cervical canal will show, on vertebral angiograms, a downward displacement of the caudal loop of the inferior posterior cerebellar artery. Also, the tonsillar branches were observed below the foramen magnum and the choroid arch was displaced downward.[21,22] The antiographic findings are not characteristic because a neoplasm will cause similar changes, although, if other evidence of an expanding lesion is absent (tumor stain), the Arnold-Chiari malformation should be considered in combination with the myelographic findings.

IV. THE DISTURBANCES OF THE NEURAL CANAL FUSION

Malformations associated with the disturbances of the neural canal fusion are initiated about the 3rd week of embryonic development. Defects of the fusion (dysrhaphia) can cause malformations of the nervous system linked to anomalies of the overlying mesenchymal tissue. The term rachischisis is commonly applied and it encompasses different types of defects. The bony defect is usually dorsal, mostly in the lumbo-sacral area (about 85%) and less in cervical or thoracic regions (approximately 10% of cases).[18,19] Ventral defects of the vertebral bodies are not often encountered.

A simple form of such defects is *spina bifida occulta* which represents a bony defect, mostly in the lumbosacral region, and which does not contain the nervous tissue. It may be covered by lipomata, pilonidal sinuses, or nevi. The bony defect is often asymptomatic, although an occasional low back pain was attributed to the spina bifida. Pathologic examinations can disclose at times a minor dysplasia of the spinal cord below the defect. Spinal *meningoceles* are a more complex type of defect that contain meninges, whereas *meningomyeloceles* include meninges and parts of the nervous tissue as well. The contents of such sacs comprise meninges with spinal nerves and portions of the spinal cord which are often dysplastic, condensed, and not easy to recognize. Deformities of the lower extremities with muscular atrophy are often connected with these malformations. Ulcerations and erosions of the skin are frequently combined with paralysis and incontinence in these patients.[18,23,24,27] An ascending leptomeningitis is not rare. Approximately 80% of the spinal meningoceles and myelomeningoceles are associated with hydrocephalus and possibly with the Arnold-Chiari malformation as mentioned above. Spinal meningoceles are less frequent than myelomeningoceles.[25,27] Diverse types of meningoceles were described in literature. Some of them, associated with Marfan's syndrome, Ehlers-Danlos syndrome, and different types of bone dysplasia, represent various dilatations of the subarachnoid space but not the true meningocele.

Some forms of true meningoceles will be briefly described. Absence of the bone on the ventral surface of the sacrum can produce an *anterior sacral meningocele*. Different clinical manifestations can be attributed to this type of meningocele including anomalies of the genitourinary and intestinal tracts, club-foot, or other musculoskeletal abnormalities. This type of meningocele should be recognized because often they form a palpable mass localized posterior to the rectum. The rectum may be displaced forward and laterally.[23,25,27] The meningocele on the rectal palpation will become tense if the patient coughs or strains due to the increase of the CSF pressure. Meningocele can be demonstrated by myelography, either with opaque or radiolucent contrast media (Figures 3 and 4). If the meningocele has a narrow neck, gas myelography, in our experience, is the method of choice because gas penetrates into the meningeal sac much easier than an insoluble contrast medium. Water-soluble contrast agents can outline the sac well even if the neck is narrow. If insoluble opaque contrast media are used, it is necessary at times to leave the contrast medium in the subarachnoid space, and keep the patient with the elevated back in the supine position for several hours in order to fill the communication between the subarachoid space and the meningocele (Figures 5 through 7).

The majority of *dorsal meningoceles,* known also as lateral meningoceles, are often linked with neurofibromatosis. They are accompanied by kyphoscoliosis, erosions of the posterior and lateral aspect of the vertebral bodies, enlargement of the foramina, destruction of the pedicles, enlargement of the spinal canal, and the presence of the soft tissue mass projecting over the spine, or lateral to the spine. The radiographic appearance of the posterior mediastinal mass, with possible changing of shape on straining, is characteristic of this type of meningocele. Myelographic examination with gas will show a free passage of oxygen from the subarachnoid space to the meningeal sac and its contents, actually, the spinal cord and nerve roots.[28] The direction of the spinal cord and nerve roots is posterior and caudad with a different degree of elongation. The neck of such a sac and its relation to the bony defect can be equally clearly demonstrated. Myelography with opaque contrast media can provide a good picture of the size and shape of the meningeal sac, although the intracavitary components may prove difficult to recognize. The penetration of the opaque medium through a narrow neck into the sac may be laborious.

In *lipomeningoceles,* the fatty lesions are demonstrated with gas myelography as densities, or as radiolucencies if the positive contrast media are used. In *postoperative meningoceles,* a large herniation of the arachnoid through an unclosed dura will occur. This type of meningocele has the tendency to grow and become larger. Small, postoperative pouches of the dura are often seen after surgery of the lumbar disk (Figure 8).[24,25,30]

V. MENINGEAL CYSTS

Meningeal cysts occur as perineural, extradural, or intradural arachnoid cysts. All three types may represent developmental malformations, although it is believed by some investigators that the origin of perineural cysts can be linked to trauma, intradural hemorrhage, or to inflammatory processes.[26,29] Some intradural cysts will cause clinical signs of spinal cord compression.[25,28] Extradural and perineural cysts, especially those in the sacral region, may induce a sciatic pain resembling that of a disk herniation (Figure 9).

Perineural cysts may occur in all parts of the spinal column. They can be multiple and bilateral, especially in the cervical area. In the sacral region, they tend to be larger in size, and bulge along the spinal nerve roots. They arise usually from the junction between the posterior roots and the dorsal ganglia. Some investigators believe that perineural cysts do not communicate with the subarachnoid space; others, however, are of the opinion that they are connected with it.[23,25,26] If the cyst is large, it may cause an erosion on the adjacent bone, usually at the S_2 to S_3 level.[23] If there is no communication between the cyst and the subarachnoid space, it is impossible to identify the cyst by means of myelography. If the connection exists, however, bilateral and multiple small cysts can show, on myelograms, a grape-like shape along the nerve roots. A perineural cyst may also cause a displacement of the caudal end of the subarachnoid space (Figure 10).[23]

Extradural meningeal cysts appear as single or double, communicating or not. They are localized more often in the dorsal region but they can be found in the lumbosacral area as well. They do not occur in the cervical region.[24,25] An extradural meningeal cyst is a gradual ballooning of the meningeal membrane at a congenitally weak point of the dura. It can have the appearance of a diverticulum of the dura. Its walls do not contain nerve fibers that are found in the perineural cyst.

Radiologic signs comprise kyphosis with different degrees of widening of the spinal canal. An incomplete obstruction of the subarachnoid space produced by the cyst can be demonstrated by means of myelography. The cyst will be filled with the insoluble opaque contrast medium if the contrast remains in the subarachnoid space, and follow-up radiographs are obtained. A complete obstruction may be present with a smooth filling defect similar to an extramedullary tumor. An increase of protein in the CSF may be disclosed with a positive Queckenstedt's test.

Arachnoid diverticula sometimes originate intradural cysts by the valve mechanism which can provoke diverticular dilatation. The arachnoid diverticula communicate freely with the subarachnoid space or otherwise act as a space-occupying lesion being magnified by the internal secretion of their walls. These types of intradural cysts are seen more commonly among younger persons, more often in the dorsal region, but they can also occur in the cervical or lumbosacral areas. Some of the cysts in the thoracic region arise from the septum posticum. There is a great difference in opinion concerning the etiology of these cysts. Radiographic findings include a certain degree of bone absorption caused by a long-lasting pressure, thinning of the pedicles, and more accentuated concavity of the dorsal surface of the vertebral bodies. The cysts related to the septum posticum may cause a compression of the spinal cord.[28,29] They are localized predominantly between T_3 and T_7. Multiple arachnoid diverticula in dorsal area are connected with this type of cyst.

Intradural arachnoid cysts are rare. Although their origin may be similar to the one of the diverticula in the dorsal area, clinically they differ because the arachnoid cyst can create a symptomatology similar to that of extramedullary tumors. It is assumed that the compression occurs due to the valve mechanism. Namely, the cyst is filled with the CSF that cannot drain.[28,29] These cysts are unilocular, they vary in size, and sometimes, they adhere to the surrounding tissues. Their walls are usually thin. True arachnoid cysts do not fill with the contrast medium and can prove difficult to distinguish, on myelograms, from neoplasms. On the other hand, it is possible to demonstrate diverticula in many patients by means of myelography. It is further assumed that the arachnoid diverticulum may lose its communication with the subarachnoid space and form a cyst, which would imply that the two conditions are actually a continuum of the same process. If the communication of the cyst permits the entrance of the contrast medium, it will be possible to demonstrate its location, nature, and relationship to the spinal cord. Gas myelography in the prone position of the patient may show clearly the filling of the cyst with oxygen.[25,28,29]

Around the nerve root, especially in the lumbar and cervical regions, the arachnoid sleeve can be wider forming a *dilated root sleeve* that is commonly seen on myelograms. Such dilated root sleeves have no clinical significance (see Chapter 7, Figures 4 and 5). If an extension originates from the root sleeve and remains in communication with the subarachnoid space through a wider or narrower neck, it is generally called *nerve root diverticulum.* Nerve root diverticula are common findings on myelograms (Figure 11). If the neck of the diverticulum becomes narrow and permits the entrance of CSF but not its exit, a nerve root cyst may form (Figure 11).[25,29]

Following lumbar laminectomy, cyst-like communications may occur in the subarachnoid space and they are known as *postoperative meningoceles, meningeal pseudocysts,* or *spurious meningoceles.*[30,31] A tear in both the arachnoid and the dura may provide the route of an egress of the CSF into the para-vertebral space. The cavity of the pseudocyst is usually lined with connective tissue. In some cases, a complete disappearance of these cysts, presumably due to fibrosis and shrinkage of the existing sac, occurred several months after surgery.[32] Postoperative defects may cause an arachnoid herniation and forming of diverticula or meningocele. Cysts located in the cervical subarachnoid space following laminectomy and dentate ligament section can be demonstrated in most cases by either negative or positive contrast myelography. However, iatrogenic meningoceles or pseudocysts in the cervical region were described without filling with the contrast medium. The cervical spinal cord can be found incarcerated in the neck of those cysts.[30-32] Postoperative or posttraumatic pseudocysts in the thoracic and lumbar regions are more common. It is assumed that they are formed due to the CSF pressure and surgical dural defect. The fluid is eventually absorbed in the beginning by the wall of the cyst, but as the connective tissue lining forms slowly, the absorption stops simultaneously, and the accumulated fluid causes a cystic dilatation.[32] These cysts, small in the beginning, can become quite large, especially in the lumbar region. Patients may complain of lumbar or thoracic radiculopathy, back pain, and occasional meningeal irritation. Myelographic examination, if the cyst if filled with contrast medium, can provide the diagnosis. Following traumas with nerve root avulsion, pseudomeningocele may develop after a longer period of time.[33] Greater frequency of lumbar traumatic meningoceles is assumed to come from the upright position and the CSF pressure which is greater in the lumbar region than in the cervical. In addition, surgery occurs more often in the lumbar region, which may be a contributing factor.[31]

VI. THE NEURENTERIC CYST

The neurenteric cyst is known under different terms such as gastrocytoma, teratoma cyst, or mediastinal cyst of the primitive digestive system.[34] The neurenteric cyst represents a developmental anomaly considered as an embryologic defect of evolution. The notochord and the endoderm are in close contact at the beginning of the embryonic evolution. Three weeks later, they separate and the notochord gives birth to the vertebral column while the endoderm forms the primitive digestive tube. If the separation is not complete, the persistence of this initial union impedes the ventral closing of the mesodermal cells that, along with the notochord, will form the spine and thus originate the communicating cyst between the spinal cord and the primitive digestive tube. These cysts are most commonly localized in the posterior mediastinum below the vertebral defect. Malformations of the vertebrae tend to be located in the lower cervical or upper thoracic area, and comprise different degrees of spinal canal widening, hemivertebrae, anterior spina bifida, scoliosis, or diastematomyelia. The cyst may be isolated or may communicate with the epidural, subdural, or subarachnoid space.[34,35] This type of cyst can cause a compression of the spinal cord.[35] Myelography will disclose a filling defect with partial or complete obstruction of the subarachnoid space. The spinal cord may be displaced laterally, and the combination of myelographic findings with multiple bony abnormalities may indicate that such type of cyst is present.[34]

VII. THE FIXED SPINAL CORD

The fixed spinal cord or "tethered" cord is not a precise pathologic term but rather a condition linked to different anomalies that prevent the ascent of the spinal cord in relation to the growth of the spinal canal. The conus of the spinal cord can be as low as the S_1 vertebra. The fixed cord is often associated with lipoma of the filum terminale, intrathecal adhesions, epidermoid, and other anomalies. In our experience, gas myelography is the procedure of choice, which usually outlines clearly the relationship between the spinal cord and the subarachnoid space. In the sagittal projection, the spinal cord is displaced dorsally. Bands of connective tissue can be occasionally recognized and thick filum terminale outlined (Figures 12 and 13).[19,20] Different clinical signs such as dysfunction of the bladder, or a variety of musculoskeletal and sensory disorders involving the lower extremities may be related to this condition. The diagnosis by means of myelography should be reached at an early stage since surgical treatment is in most cases indicated.

Different additional anomalies can involve the spinal canal, either as single pathologic entities, or in combination with other congenital malformations.[18,19,36] Dermal sinuses seen in the lumbosacral region are related to epidermoid, teratoma, and dermoid cysts. Meningitis or abscess formation can be referred to the presence of dermal sinuses. In the absent cervical pedicle syndrome, Pantopaque® myelography may demonstrate at the level of the bony malformation two nerve roots leaving the cervical cord usually encircled in one meningeal sleeve.[12] In the duplication of the posterior vertebral arch, a compression of the spinal cervical cord may ensue.[12]

The second sac is an acquired anomaly related to multiple lumbar punctures. It will be mentioned here because it can occasionally simulate some meningeal congenital anomalies.[37] Following the insertion of the needle into the subarachnoid space, a certain amount of CSF will accumulate between the meningeal sheaths. An extensive space may be formed as mentioned in the above text. A relatively wide separation of the dura from the arachnoid and the further accumulation of the CSF will cause an abundant reflux of the CSF, although the bevel of the needle is in the subdural space. If a contrast medium is injected, two separate accumulations may be visualized: one in the subarachnoid, and the other in the subdural space. In the anteroposterior view, the subdural collection of the contrast medium appears accumulated on both sides of the subarachnoid space. In the lateral view, the two collections of the contrast agent can be seen distinctly separated. The subdural collection has generally a streaked configuration, and it does not spill into the intracranial cisterns.[37]

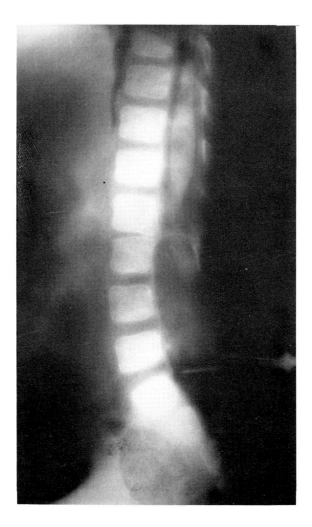

FIGURE 1.   On this gas myelogram is an unusually wide lumbosacral spinal canal and arachnoid sac. The spinal cord is stretched and fixed by a spicule of bone at L_3 level. At L_5 a soft tissue mass is recognizable extending into a meningocele. At surgery diastomyelia was found with a lipomeningocele. (Patient referred from the Clinic of Neurology, University of Geneva.)

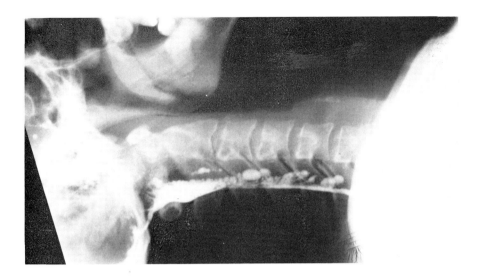

FIGURE 2. A female patient, 50 years old, had developed progressive signs of spinal cord compression. On admission, ataxia and nystagmus were especially prominent. Pantopaque® myelogram in the supine lateral position shows a bilobulated defect above C_1. The cisterna magna appears flattened. The spinal cord is displaced ventrally. The contrast medium outlines the posterior subarachnoid compartment. On the basis of this myelographic examination, and in general with myelography alone, it is difficult to differentiate an Arnold-Chiari malformation from a tumor in the upper cervical region. At surgery, the diagnosis of the Arnold-Chiari malformation was confirmed.

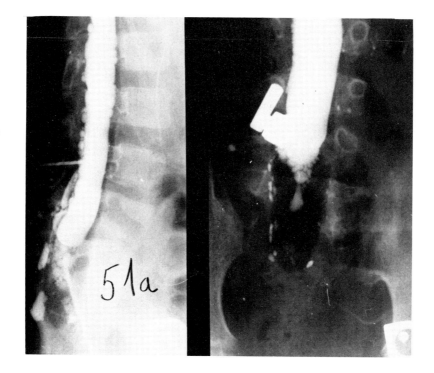

A

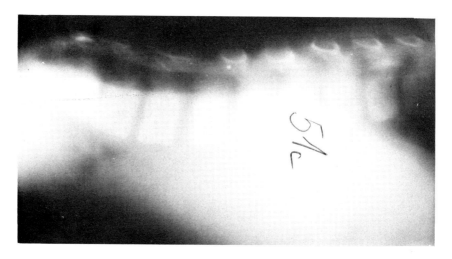

B

FIGURE 3(A).   The double contrast myelogram (oxygen and Pantopaque®) of a 3½-year-old girl demonstrates a wide arachnoid sac in the lumbosacral region and a stretched spinal cord to L₄ level. (B) The additional gas myelogram performed two weeks later shows a meningocele. The spinal cord appears compressed. At surgery, a lipoma was disclosed in the meningocele, and the spinal cord pulled downwards. (Courtesy of Department of Radiology, Johns Hopkins Hospital, Baltimore, Md.)

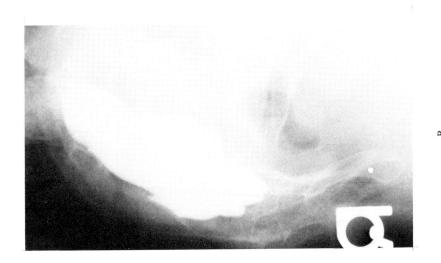

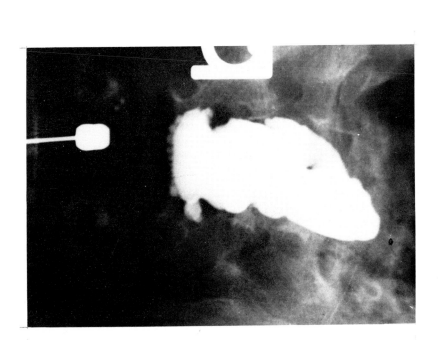

A

B

FIGURE 4(A and B). Pantopaque® myelograms disclose a large anterior sacral meningocele. (Courtesy of Department of Radiology, Johns Hopkins Hospital, Baltimore, Md.)

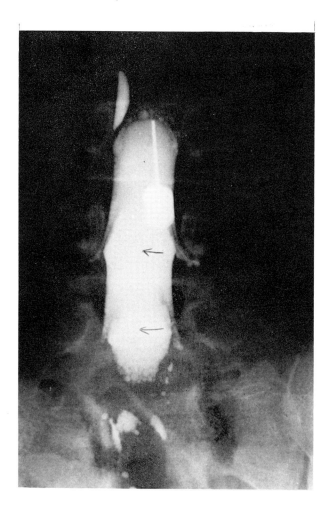

FIGURE 5. Pantopaque® myelogram demonstrates a lumbosacral meningocele with a stretched and compressed spinal cord (arrows). Some gas was injected into the arachnoid sac where the presence of a lipoma was disclosed. Note the position of the nerve roots. (Courtesy Dr. G. B. Udvarhelyi and Department of Radiology, Johns Hopkins Hospital, Baltimore, Md.)

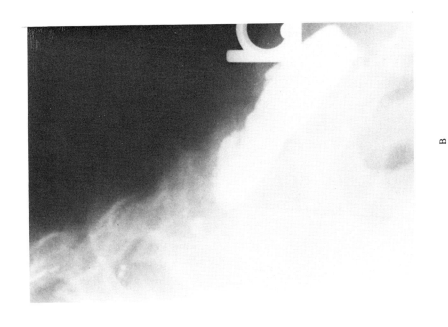

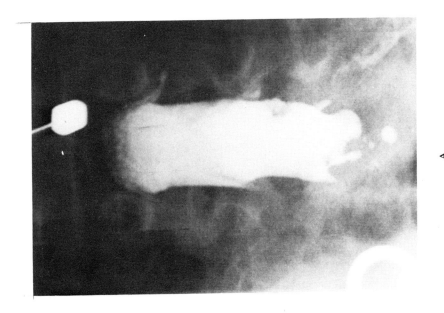

B

A

FIGURE 6(A and B). Large sacral meningocele. The spinal cord appears outlined almost to the level of L_5, with the emerging nerves. The patient is seen in an upright posture to obtain a complete filling of the arachnoid sac. (Courtesy of Dr. G. B. Udvarhelyi and Department of Radiology, Johns Hopkins Hospital, Baltimore, Md.)

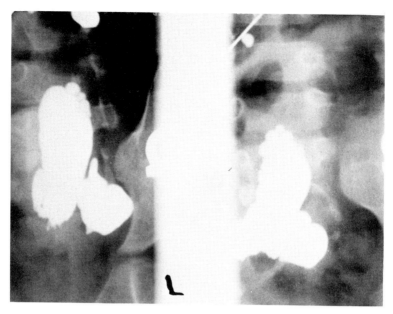

FIGURE 7.   A double sac of a sacral meningocele connected with a rather wide neck can be seen on this oblique myelogram. (Courtesy Dr. G. B. Udvarhelyi and Department of Radiology, Johns Hopkins Hospital, Baltimore, Md.)

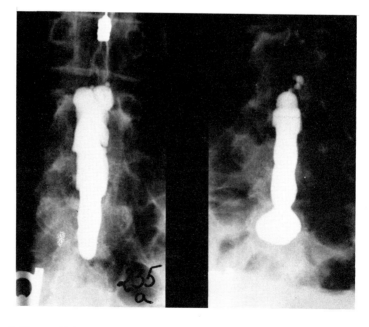

FIGURE 8.   A 49-year-old female patient had spinal fusion at L_3 level 9 years earlier. She gradually developed back and left leg pain with tingling. The neurological evaluation indicated the possibility of a new disk herniation at L_4 to L_5 level. Lumbar myelogram shows irregular margins of the arachnoid sac and right side obliteration of the meningeal sleeves at the level of previous fusion. These changes were interpreted as signs of postoperative adhesions. A large arachnoid cyst is well filled with Pantopaque® in the upright posture. At surgery the myelographic findings were confirmed. The pressure by the cyst on the nerve root and the adhesions were the cause of the clinical symptomatology.

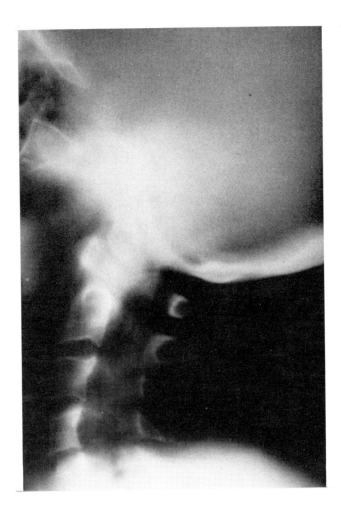

A

FIGURE 9.   The patient, a 36-year-old female, was admitted with signs of cervical radiculomyelopathy following neck injury. Two myelographies were performed. (A) Gas myelogram of the cervical area demonstrates the escape of gas into a large meningeal sac which could not be well interpreted. (B) Pantopaque® myelogram shows an accumulation of the contrast medium in the lower cervical region. A partial obstruction was present at C_7. (C and D) In two different accentuated oblique positions the contrast medium moved cranially and the leakage of Pantopaque® is seen at the level of left C_5 to C_3 nerve roots. (E) In the lateral projection, the contrast medium is divided into two layers. It fills a large cyst that communicates with the subarachnoid and subdural space. At surgery, a large arachnoid cyst was found at C_3 to C_6 level covered by the dura.

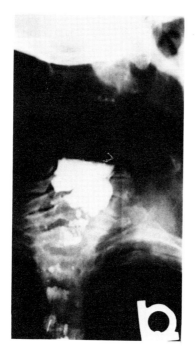
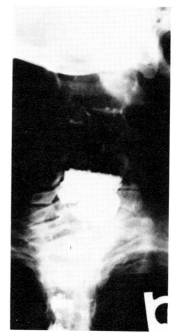

FIGURE 9B.

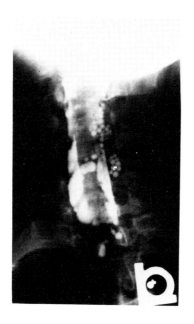
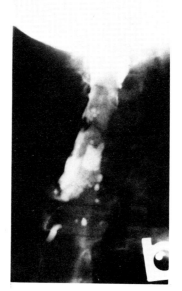

FIGURE 9C.

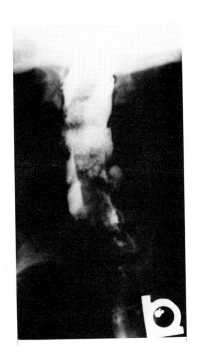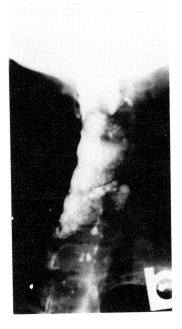

FIGURE 9D.

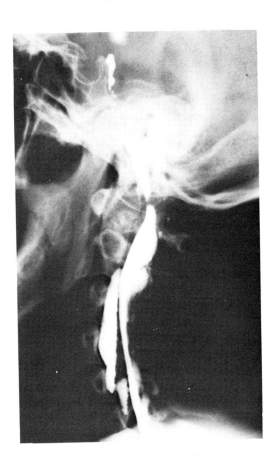

FIGURE 9E.

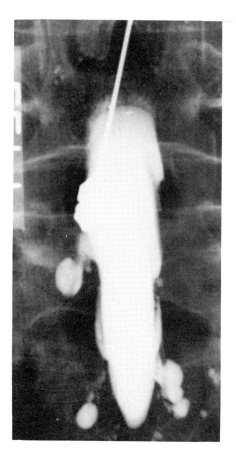

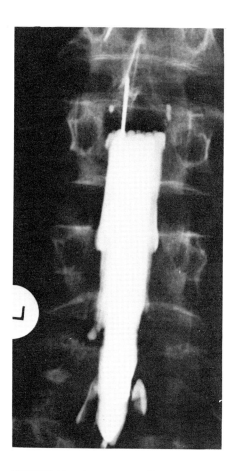

FIGURE 10. Pantopaque® myelogram in the lumbosacral area reveals larger and smaller perineural cysts. The nerves are seen transsecting the cysts. In the right sacral region multiple small communicating cysts surrounding a nerve appear in a grape-like shape.

FIGURE 11. A nerve root diverticula and a few small cysts are visible in the lumbosacral segment on this Pantopaque® myelogram. The nerves are encircled by dilated meninges. At the right L_4 to L_5 level a nerve root is compressed by a disk herniation and also enlarged by edema.

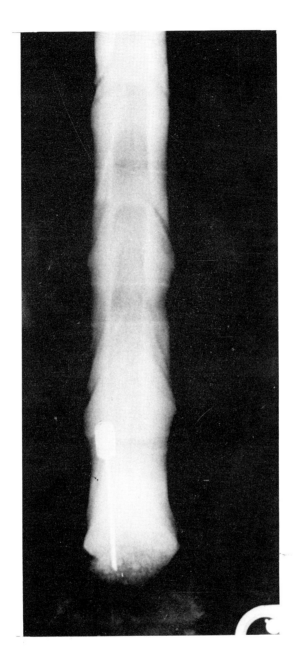

A

FIGURE 12(A). Pantopaque® myelogram, anteroposterior view, in this 17-year-old male patient shows a
stretched spinal cord ("tethered" cord) extending below S_1
level. The nerve roots are prominent. (B) In an almost erect
posture a large sacral meninogocele is delineated. (C) Lateral projection of the sacral area demonstrates the full size
of the meningocele, a large nerve root, and the filum terminale. The surgery confirmed the myelographic findings.
(Courtesy of Dr. F. Hodges, Department of Radiology,
Johns Hopkins Hospital, Baltimore, Md.)

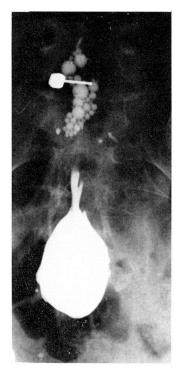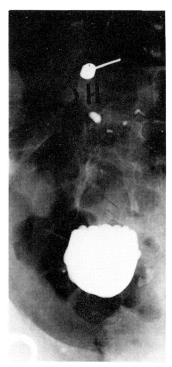

FIGURE 12B.

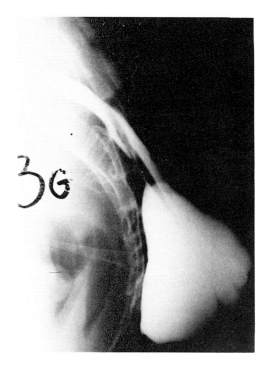

FIGURE 12C.

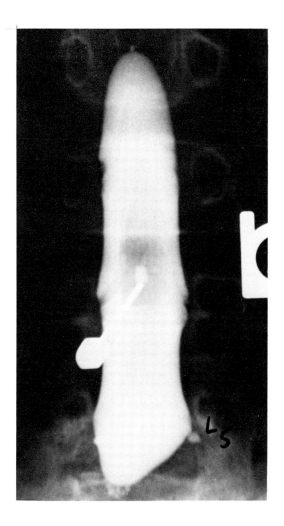

A

FIGURE 13(A). Pantopaque® myelograms outline a wide lumbosacral subarachnoid space with a stretched and fixed spinal cord at L_5. The nerves are seen leaving the spinal cord. (B) In oblique positions the size of this lipo-meningocele is well demonstrated. The stretched spinal cord with its nerves is also visualized. (C) In the upright, prone position of the patient the meningocele is apparent. (Courtesy Dr. G. B. Udvarhelyi and Department of Radiology, Johns Hopkins Hospital, Baltimore, Md.)

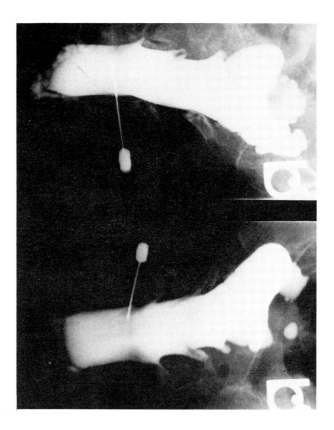

FIGURE 13C.

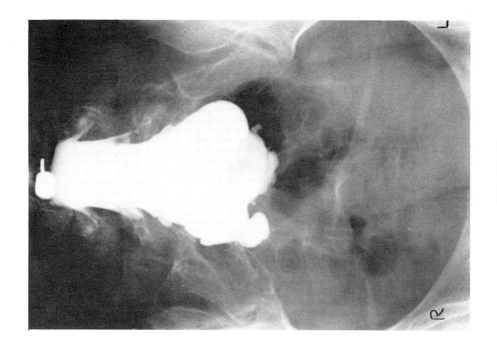

FIGURE 13B.

REFERENCES

1. **Weil, A. and Matthews, W. B.,** Duplication of the spinal cord, with spina bifida and syringomyelia, *Arch. Pathol.,* 20, 882, 1935.
2. **Lichtenstein, W.,** *Syringomyelia, Hydromyelia and Pseudosyringomyelia,* W. B. Saunders, Philadelphia, 1949.
3. **Bremer, J. L.,** Dorsal intestinal fistula; accessory neurenteric canal; diastematomyelia, *Arch. Pathol.,* 54, 132, 1952.
4. **Seaman, W. B. and Schwartz, H. G.,** Diastematomyelia in adults, *Radiology,* 70, 692, 1958.
5. **James, C. C. M. and Lassman, L. P.,** Diastematomyelia, *Arch. Dis. Child.,* 33, 536, 1958.
6. **James, C. C. M. and Lassman, L. P.,** Diastematomyelia, *Arch. Dis. Child.,* 39, 125, 1964.
7. **Sarwar, M. and Kelly, P. J.,** Adult diastematomyelia, *Spine,* 2, 60, 1977.
8. **Herren, R. Y. and Edwards, J. E.,** Diplomyelia (duplication of the spinal cord), *Arch. Pathol.,* 30, 1203, 1940.
9. **Epstein, B. S.,** *The Spine,* 4th ed., Lea & Febiger, Philadelphia, 1976, chap. 8.
10. **Marclay, J. G., Bessler, W., and Loher, E.,** Radiologische Zeichen einer Diastematomyelie, *Radiol. Clin. Biol.,* 41, 264, 1972.
11. **Pigault, P., Pouliquen, J. C., Guyonvarch, G., and Durand, Y.,** Quatre cas de diastematomyelie, *Revue Chir. Orthopedique Reparatrice Appareil Moteur Paris,* 58, 33, 1972.
12. **Shapiro, R.,** *Myelography,* 3rd ed., Year Book Medical Publishers, Chicago, 1975, chap. 11.
13. **Arnold, J.,** Myelocyste. Transposition von Gewebskeimen und Sympodie, *Beitr. Path. Anat. Allg. Pathol.,* 16, 1, 1894.
14. **Chiari, H.,** Über Veränderungen des Kleinhirns, des Pons und der Meddula oblongata in Folge von Kongenitalen Hydrocephalie des Grosshirns, *Denkschr. d. k. Akad. Wissensch. Mathem. Nat. KL.,* 63, 71, 1896.
15. **Goldstein, F. and Kepes, J. J.,** The relationship of the Arnold-Chiari malformation to lumbar meningomyeloceles. An experimental study, *Proc. Fifth Inter. Congr. Neuropathology,* Excerpta Medica Foundation, 734, 1966.
16. **Robertson, E. G.** *Pneumoencephalography,* 2nd ed., Charles C Thomas, Springfield, Ill., 1967, chap. 29.
17. **Russell, D. S. and Donald, C.,** The mechanism of internal hydrocephalus in spina bifida, *Brain,* 58, 203, 1935.
18. **Norman, R. M.,** Malformations of the nervous system, birth injury, and diseases of early life, in *Greenfield's Neuropathology,* 2nd ed., Blackwood, W., McMenemy, W. H., Meyer, A., Norman, R.M., and Russel, D. S., Eds., Williams & Wilkins, Baltimore, 1966.
19. **Hugues, J. T.,** *Pathology of the Spinal Cord,* W. B. Saunders, Philadelphia, 1978, chap. 2.
20. **Decker, K.,** *Klinische Neuroradiologie,* Georg Thieme Verlag, Stuttgart, 1960, chap. 7.
21. **Krayenbrihl, H. A. and Yasargil, M. G.,** *Cerebral Angiography,* J. B. Lippincott, Philadelphia, 1968, chap. 2.
22. **Newton, T. H. and Potts, D. G.,** *Angiography,* Vol. 2 (Part 12), C. V.Mosby, St. Louis, 1974, chap. 68, 1766.
23. **Seaman, W. B.,** Myelography appearance of sacral cysts, *J. Neurosurg.,* 13, 88, 1956.
24. **Jacobs, L. G., Smith, J. K., and Van Horn, P. S.,** Meylographic demonstration of cysts of spinal membrane, *Radiology,* 62, 215, 1954.
25. **Lombardi, G. and Morello, G.,** Congenital cysts of the spinal membranes and roots, *Br. J. Radiol.,* 36, 197, 1963.
26. **Tarlov, I. M.,** Perineural cysts of spinal nerve roots, *Arch. Neurol. Psychiatry,.* 40, 1067, 1938.
27. **Hertzog, E., Bamberger-Bozo, C., and Rougerie, J.,** Les Myélo-méningocèles, *Ann. Radiol.,* 14, 627, 1971.
28. **Sang, U. K., Baloh, R. W., and Weingarten, S.,** Intradural arachnoid cysts presenting with cord compression, *Bull. Los Angeles Neurol. Soc.,* 37, 178, 1972.
29. **Vyhnanek, L., Zeman, M., and Trivedi, R. M.,** Die Radikulären und subduralen Zysten im peridurographische Bild, *Fortschr. Röntgenstr.,* 116, 160, 1972.
30. **Kim, Y. W., DeBoer Unger, J., and Grinsell, P. J.,** Post-operative pseudodiverticula (spurious meningoceles) of the cervical subarachnoid space, *Acta Radiol. Diagn.,* 15, 16, 1974.
31. **Cobb, C., III, and Ehni, G.,** Herniation of the spinal cord into an iatrogenic meningocele, *J. Neurosurg.,* 39, 533, 1973.
32. **Miller, P. R. and Elder, F. W.,** Meningeal pseudocysts (meningocele spurious) following laminectomy: report of ten cases, *J. Bone J. Surg.,* 50A, 268, 1968.
33. **Keim, H. A.,** Cord paralysis following injection into traumatic cervical meningocele: complication of stellate gauglion block, *N.Y. Med. J.,* 70, 2115, 1970.

34. **Gimeno, A., Lopez, F., Figuera, D., and Rodrigo, L.,** Neuroentheric cyst, *Neuroradiology,* 3, 167, 1972.
35. **Dorsey, J. F. and Tabrisky, J.,** Intraspinal and mediastinal foregut cyst compressing the spinal cord. Report of a case, *J. Neurosurg.,* 24, 562, 1966.
36. **Sorensen, B. F. and Wirthlin, A. J.,** Redundant nerve roots of the cauda equina, *Surg. Neurol.,* 3, 177, 1975.
37. **Rogoff, E. E., Deck, M. D. F., and D'Angio, G.,** The second sac, *Am. J. Roentgenol.,* 120, 568, 1974.

Chapter 9

INJURIES TO THE SPINAL CORD AND MENINGES

I. INTRODUCTION

Trauma may be produced by mechanical kinetic energy transmitted to the vertebral column and its contents as an acceleration force that causes fractures, lacerations, contusions, hemorrhages, and vascular lesions. Nonmechanical forces such as pressure, ultrasound, laser, and electromagnetic radiation may also transfer energy to the spinal cord in different ways and cause trauma. Injuries that occur during birth represent a separate pathologic entity that will not be discussed in this text.

Mechanical forces can have different effects. They can cause, for instance, a *blunt impact,* and the injury produced depends on the area of impact, velocity, mass, and whether the spinal column is fixed or movable. If the dura remains intact, the injury is considered closed, or open if the bony structures are fractured and the meninges lacerated. The *penetrating wounds* are induced by objects such as bullets, knives, flying glass, or metal fragments. Such objects may penetrate the bony structures of the spinal canal, dura, leptomeninges, and the spinal cord. The type of trauma produced under these conditions depends upon the shape of the object, its sharpness, and velocity of penetration. Penetrating wounds caused by knife are usually lateral of the midline because the spinal laminae prevent the sharp edge of the knife from entering directly from behind. Thus, hemisection of the spinal cord is common. Sometimes, both posterior columns can be severed. The damage caused ranges from small lesions to a complete transsection and the amount of hemorrhage will depend upon the injury to the blood vessels. Bone fragments or displacements of the bony structures may also cause penetrating injuries. The impact can create a sudden flexion, or extension of the neck associated with the compression of blood vessels, protrusion of intervertebral disks, and bone fragments, and direct tears and contusions of the spinal cord can also take place* (Figures 1 and 2).[1,2,25]

Although the spinal cord is relatively fixed by septa and suspended in the CSF that has a specific gravity close to that of the nervous tissue, the cord may be accelerated by the action of a force. Lesions directly beneath the impact are called "coup", and those on the opposite side to the impact are referred as "contrecoup". Impacts at obtuse angles may generate angular acceleration or torsion of the spinal cord with shearing stresses and tearing.[1,2] The penetrating objects provoke direct laceration of the tissue with disruption, hemorrhage, and necrosis. They open, in addition, a smaller or larger wound through which infectious agents may enter the spinal canal and cord. In the presence of injured and dead tissues, ideal conditions exist for inflammation and abcess formation.[25]

Extradural compression of the spinal cord can be caused by disk herniation or vertebral bony dislocations with or without fractures. Later the callus formation around the fracture site may also compress the spinal cord.[2]

Concussion originating from a sudden blow is probably the least noxious and easily reversible disturbance of the spinal cord function. Contusion, induced by a crushing injury to the spinal cord, may produce lesions of different severity. It can provoke hemorrhage and edema involving several segments above and below the site of injury.

---

* All figures appear following text.

The hemorrhage usually occurs in the central part of the spinal cord and may expand, dissecting the cord longitudinally along the fiber tracts. High velocity bullets can produce compression waves that cause contusion and edema of the spinal cord at a distance from the lesion. Laceration and crushing may create in the spinal cord local softening, hemorrhage, and liquefaction. Following the trauma, adhesions of the meninges often result in dense and extensive scars associated with circulatory and ischemic disturbances. Further on, a cyst may form at the site of the lesion, and secondary ascending and descending degeneration may occur within the tissue of the spinal cord. Posttraumatic cysts are found in the shape of a syrinx and, occasionally, a progressive syringomyelia may follow.[2] Lesions in the spinal cord resulting from a trauma will be recovered by the proliferation of connective tissue.[25]

II. RADIOLOGIC ASPECTS OF TRAUMA

The radiologic aspects of the most common sequelae of the injuries to the spinal cord and surrounding meningeal sheaths can be summarized in the following way.

A. Epidural Hematoma

Epidural hematoma is usually venous in origin and probably caused through tearing of small veins (Batson's veins) due to an increased pressure by impact or penetrating objects.[2] Epidural hematoma is generated by injuries of different severity, and it is seen in association with even minor traumas. It should be mentioned that an extradural hematoma may also occur spontaneously in connection with anticoagulant therapy, in infections, and in conjunction with vascular neoplasms.[3,26] The site of an extradural hemorrhage is mostly in the dorsal epidural space which is wider. The cross-table lateral myelograms in the prone position, or lateral tomograms if gas myelography is used, are often decisive for the diagnosis. The compression of the spinal cord disclosed on myelography with opaque or lucent contrast media will vary depending upon the quantity of epidural extravasation. The ventral displacement of the compressed cord usually extends over several segments. Due to the compression, the cord in the prone position appears to be wider. This misleading appearance may simulate the myelographic signs of intramedullary hematoma or edema. If the epidural hematoma is extended more laterally, it will cause a displacement of the spinal cord and nerves to the opposite side. In case of severe compression of the spinal cord, an obstruction of the subarachnoid space may occur and a complete block will be demonstrated on myelograms with opaque contrast media.[4] Often, gas can bypass the obstruction and outline the extent of the extradural hematoma. After a period of time, extradural hematomas may become encapsulated or substituted with a fibrous and dense scarring tissue producing, mostly in the lumbar region, myelographic signs of a nonspecific epidural expanding lesion (Figures 3, 4, 5, and 6).

A posttraumatic epidural hematoma should be differentiated from an acute spontaneous hemorrhage that occurs abruptly and is characterized clinically by a sudden severe pain that may be associated with radicular distribution. Later, a progressive loss of function of variable severity can follow.[3] Acute epidural hematoma, in addition to back and radicular pain, can cause paresis and urinary retention. Paresis may progress to paraplegia or tetraplegia within a short period of time. An immediate diagnosis followed by surgical decompression is necessary, except in a very rare spontaneous remission. In the region of a cauda equina, the hemorrhage may become encapsulated and a chronic hematoma may simulate the clinical signs produced by an intervertebral disk herniation.[3,5-7] The spontaneous epidural hematoma usually occurs in the thoracic area, although it can involve other regions of the spinal column, as well. The presentation of fractures and dislocations of the vertebrae may be of assistance to differentiate a posttraumatic epidural hematoma from those of other origins. Equally important is the clinical information that may reveal that the patient was treated for hemophilia, leukemia, or other blood dyscrasias, or has been receiving anticoagulant therapy.[2,6,26]

B. Subdural Hematoma

Subdural hematoma following injuries to the spine and meninges is a rare pathologic finding.[2] It can occur in an acute or subacute fashion, and may appear associated with lumbar puncture or some blood dyscrasias, especially hemophilia.[6] The myelographic findings are not characteristic. They show a complete or partial obstruction of the subarachnoid space and a compression and displacement of the spinal cord in the ventro, dorsal, or lateral direction.[6-8] A subdural hematoma can be partially or completely encapsulated and in this case it can impose compression of the spinal cord.[8] Adhesions that form obliterate the fissure between the arachnoid and the dura. They can also extend into the subarachnoid space and involve the pia.[8] It may be difficult to distinguish such pathologic changes on myelographic studies from other pathologic processes of the subarachnoid space.

A subdural hematoma following back injury is usually linked to spinal pain, fever, meningism, paralyses, and hematorrhachis. If myelography is carried out, the lumbar puncture may be difficult and, often, it is necessary to inject the contrast medium into the cisterna magna.

C. Subarachnoid Hemorrhage

Subarachnoid hemorrhage caused by penetrating wounds is often combined with epidural bleeding and spinal cord lesions. This type of hemorrhage should be differentiated from the spontaneous subarachnoid hemorrhage which is rare and occurs mainly in male adults. In addition, the subarachnoid hemorrhage can be associated with a number of different conditions such as vascular malformations, aneurysms, blood dyscrasias, coarctation of the aorta, inflammatory diseases, nerve root avulsion, and neoplasms. This variety of different, underlying pathologic processes which may be the origin of subarachnoid hemorrhage is fully described in literature.[4,10,25] If myelography is required, a lumbar puncture will show the presence of fresh blood in the CSF. The fluid in a less acute situation can be xanthochromic. Therefore, before the instillation of the opaque contrast medium, the performance of myelography should be reconsidered. However, in the presence of clinical signs such as severe, sudden headache, neck pain with rigidity, opisthotonos if the hemorrhage occured in the cervical area, or abrupt severe low back pain if the hemorrhage is mainly in the lumbar region, myelography should be carried out. We did not encounter difficulties with the injection of the positive or negative contrast media under these circumstances. It is expected that the utilization of Metrizamide® may solve the problem of myelography in the presence of subarachnoid hemorrhage. A smaller amount of the opaque contrast medium is ordinarily injected without being later removed from the subarachnoid space. An injection of about 6 cc will provide the information regarding the state of the subarachnoid space. The myelogram can demonstrate a complete or partial obstruction of the subarachnoid space depending upon the involvement of the spinal cord. If the origin of the hemorrhage is related to a tumor such as ependymoma, neurofibroma, hemangioblastoma, or occasionally meningioma, the myelogram will supply additional information concerning these space-occupying lesions.[10] The evaluation of standard radiographs may disclose the presence of fractures and dislocations, and it can facilitate the differential diagnosis of a posttraumatic subarachnoid hemorrhage.

The extradural, subdural, and subarachnoid hemorrhages are often intermixed in penetrating wounds of the spine and cannot be differentiated by means of myelography (Figure 7). The lesion of the spinal cord that accompanies this type of bleeding is common and it will complicate the radiologic diagnostic evaluation.[2] Furthermore, blunt trauma can cause a formation of an extradural cyst that may communicate through a fistula with the subarachnoid space.[9,25] Myelography will show filling of the cyst with the contrast medium. If this communication does not exist, a deformity of the subarachnoid space may indicate the presence of an epidural space-occupying lesion. On very rare occasions is a cyst formed in the subdural space.[11-13]

D. Hematomyelia and Edema

Hematomyelia and edema cause swelling of the spinal cord that becomes rounded and tense within the meninges, and the subarachnoid and subdural spaces may be obliterated. The cord edema extends the seat of an acute traumatic damage and the involved area often has the shape of a spindle. Apart from edema, an accumulation of blood may occur in the spinal cord associated with hyperemia and venous stasis. However, there are some doubts as to whether injury causes true hematomyelia. It is mostly at the site of the spinal cord trauma that the disintegration of the nervous tissue occurs. The trauma at this location more often produces pulping and a hemorrhagic infarction than a large intramedullary hemorrhage characteristic of hematomyelia and seen more frequently in relation to angiomatous malformation and hemorrhagic diathesis.[2,25,26]

About 3 weeks after the trauma to the spinal cord, the acute changes subside and an intermediate period begins characterized by the disappearance of edema and absorption of the necrotic tissue and blood. The presence of astrocytic gliosis further on leads to scar formation, the extension of which depends upon the degree of damage.[25] Chronic posttraumatic changes take place after a longer period of time, occasionally 5 to 10 years. They are marked by a traumatic scar and the presence of collagenous connective tissue which causes a fusion between the meninges and the spinal cord. The longitudinal cavity within the spinal cord, which replaces the area of hemorrhagic necrosis of the acute stage of the injury, can later have a glial and connective tissue lining that forms a thick wall. A posttraumatic syringomyelia may develop with signs of an upward expansion of the spinal cord lesion occurring after a longer period of a stable neurologic state following the initial injury.[14-16] The newly developed neurological signs may have a rapid onset. In the majority of cases, traumatic syringomyelia represents an upward cavitation starting from the site of the original injury. The downward cavitation, if it happens, does not bring forward clinical signs. The mechanism of the development of the posttraumatic syrinx has not been fully explained. There is a possibility that a communication is formed between the syrinx and the subarachnoid space close to the posterior root entry.[2]

The clinical symptomatology of a spinal cord injury will depend upon its location and the extent of the damage. Paralysis below the lesion may develop with hypalgesia and hypesthesia. The use of myelography in severe spinal cord injuries should be considered in relation to the clinical signs and possible injuries to the bony structures of the spine. The myelographic technique will depend equally upon these factors. Often, a suboccipital or cervical instillation of the contrast medium is necessary. Myelography in trauma should be carefully planned not to cause further damage to the cord by dislocation of the fractured bony components. The choice of the contrast medium may be important. On many occasions, we used gas myelography. Metrizamide® may prove to be more adequate than Pantopaque® myelography in spinal cord injuries.

In the acute stage of a trauma, the myelogram shows an enlarged cord in the cervical or thoracic area with irregular contours and pronounced, swollen nerve roots (Figures 8 and 9). In extensive cord dilatation, a complete obstruction to the flow of the contrast medium will be present. Various pathologic processes that occur in the injury of the spinal cord cannot always be distinguished on the basis of myelography. It should be mentioned that a hemorrhage of the spinal cord may originate in association with different diseases, especially hemophilia. The history of injury and the eventual presence of dislocation and fragmentation of vertebrae will point to the diagnosis. In the course of myelographic examination, attention should be paid to the nerve roots that may be severed as well as the dentate ligaments. The leakage of the contrast medium can be detected if the injury to the spinal cord is combined with a tear of the meninges. The posttraumatic spinal cord swelling is associated quite frequently with a certain degree of damage to the meninges and possibly with subarachnoid or epidural hematomas. In the stable clinical period that follows an injury of the spine, myelography may disclose adhesions or a localized enlargement of the spinal cord brought about by the presence of a syrinx. If the syrinx is extensive, the spinal cord will have a diffusely swollen appearance, commonly clearly demonstrated on gas myelography (Figures 6 and 10). Myelography can disclose extensive adhesions causing obliteration of the subarachnoid space. Multiple filling defects can be seen on myelograms with the cord completely imbedded in thick adhesions, compressed, and attached to the anterior or posterior wall of the spinal canal (Figure 11). A lateral attachment of the spinal cord can occur combined with a tear of the dentate ligament on the opposite side. In 120 posttraumatic myelograms that we evaluated, the changes involving the spinal canal and cord varied from barely noticeable radiologic signs of adhesions to a localized syrinx, diffuse posttraumatic syringomyelia, and adhesions causing partial obstructions (Figures 12 and 13).

E. Nerve Root Avulsion

The nerve root avulsion is connected with severe traumas, and usually occurs in the cervical region although it can also appear in the lumbosacral area. The avulsion of the root represents the severance of the nerve combined with the meningeal tear. Fractures and bony dislocations of the vertebrae can be present too. If the arm is in a forced adduction at the impact, the nerve roots at the C_5 and C_6 levels will be exposed to the injury and a paralysis of Erb-Duchenne type will occur. On the other hand, if the arm is in abduction, the lower cervical and the upper thoracic nerve roots could be involved. The resulting paralysis is mostly of the Klumpke type.[18] Occasionally, when the first thoracic nerve is injured, Horner's syndrome may develop. If an opaque contrast medium is injected into the subarachnoid space, the myelography will show a characteristic leakage of Pantopaque® into one or more pockets directed downward and laterally. (Figures 13 and 14). The size of these pockets varies considerably. In small lacerations, the leakage may be barely visible and therefore its detection on myelograms may prove difficult. The shape of the pockets appears very irregular. The radiolucency of the nerve root is absent, a characteristic feature not seen in diverticula (Figure 15).[17,18,21]

The avulsion of the cervical nerve roots provoked by traction injuries to the shoulder region is by far more common than the traumatic avulsion of the nerve roots in the lumbar and sacral regions.[19,20] Assumably, the resistance and stability of the bony structures of the pelvis protect the nerve roots that are less susceptible to stretching in case of injury. Even in traumas of the pelvis, the avulsion of the nerve roots occurs in approximately 0.41 to 1.2% of cases.[19] Injuries caused to the S_1 and S_2 nerve roots resulting in motor deficit, pain, and dysesthesia or hypesthesiaare usually connected to transverse or other types of fractures of the sacrum and differ from the nerve root avulsion. The nerve root avulsion in this area is linked to pelvic trauma causing separation of sacroiliac joint. This separation permits a considerable mobility of the bony structures that normally protect the nerve roots. A forceful shearing linked to sacroiliac joint separation may cause root tearing. It is possible that a violent flexion and abduction of the hip may produce the avulsion of the L_4 nerve root. It seems that the nerve root avulsion occurs close to the intervertebral foramen.[22-24]

In case of lumbosacral nerve root avulsion, myelography will disclose a picture very similar to the one in the cervical area. Wide and often irregular outpouchings of the subarachnoid space around the affected nerve roots will be demonstrated, yet the nerve root itself will not be outlined. These cyst-like formations are results of the tearing of the arachnoid and eventually of the dura which follow the nerve root to its exit.

The nerve root meningocele may have a similar appearance on myelograms as the nerve root avulsion. However, the nerve root is seen as a linear radiolucency in the meningocele. The root meningocele may have a relatively narrow neck and a wide sac-like ending. The meningoceles are often multiple and can appear on both sides of the subarachnoid space. These cysts are usually asymptomatic and not related to the trauma, although some were held responsible for the development of the sciatic syndrome.[20,24] In the case of nerve root avulsion, often a severe neurologic deficit in the affected dermatome will clearly differentiate this lesion from a nerve root meningocele. In addition, the appearance of flaccid paralysis, and later the development of evident muscle wasting is common in the nerve root avulsion. Most often, the motor and sensory deficits are both equally severe in the nerve root avulsion. These clinical features distinguish the nerve root avulsion from different widenings of the meningeal nerve root sleeves seen on myleograms.[22-24]

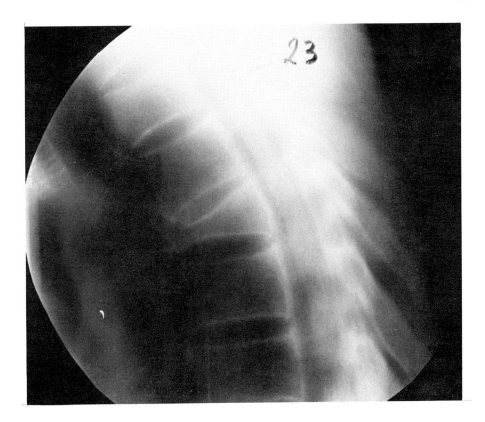

FIGURE 1. Gas myelogram showing a fracture of Th$_6$ vertebra in the thoracic area. There are no signs of spinal cord compression. The epidural space at Th$_5$ to Th$_6$ levels looks wider indicating the presence of circumscribed epidural bleeding. (Patient referred from the Department of Neurology, University of Geneva).

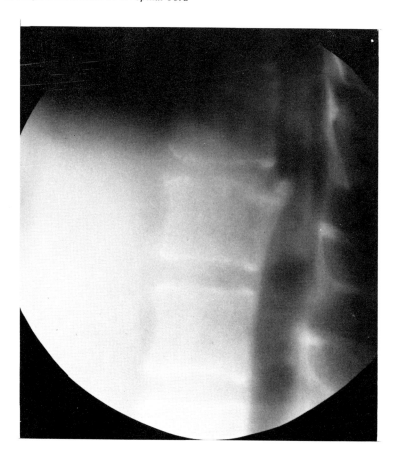

FIGURE 2.   The fracture of L_1 vertebra in the lumbar region, as well as the ventral compression of the subarachnoid space and spinal cord, are disclosed by this gas myelogram. The radiolucent line along the dorsal surface of the vertebral body represents an epidural hematoma. (Patient referred from the Clinic of Neurosurgery, University of Geneva). At surgery, a decompression was performed and the radiologic findings confirmed.

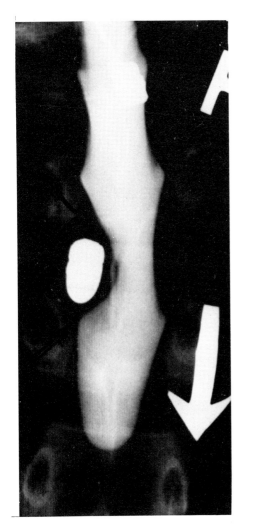
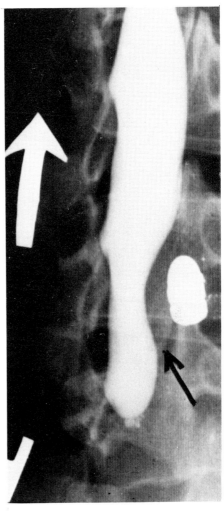

A

B

FIGURE 3. Pantopaque® myelography performed following a lumbar bullet wound. (A) Epidural compression of the subarachnoid space due to a large extradural hematoma and the bullet. (B) The contrast medium moves freely in the cranial direction in an otherwise large canal. (C) Lateral projection shows the relationship between the bullet and the subarachnoid space and the spinal column at the level of L_3. At surgery, a large epidural hematoma was evacuated as well as the bullet. (Courtesy of the Department of Radiology, Johns Hopkins Hospital, Baltimore, Md.).

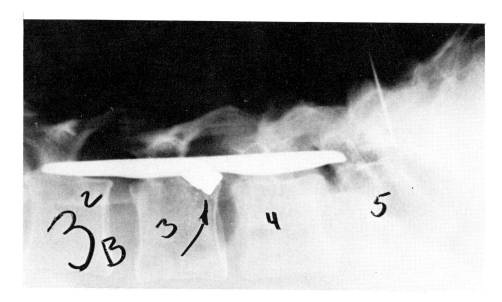

FIGURE 3C

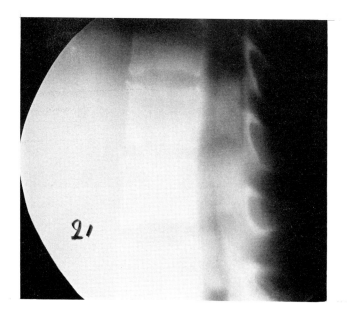

A

FIGURE 4(A).   Midline gas myelogram represents a wide epidural hematoma extending from L_2 vertebra caudally. The conus of the spinal cord and the subarachnoid space are compressed ventrally. The patient had received a penetrating wound at L_2 by a bullet a few hours prior to myelography. (B) Gas myelogram obtained 2 mm to the right of the midline (the distance between adjacent objective planes on polytomograph was 2 mm) demonstrates the extent of the spinal cord and subarachnoid space compression. (C) The sacral area gas myelogram reveals the bullet lodging in the subarachnoid space among the nerves which are seen as fine linear radiolucencies. The bullet was rolling freely in the lower subarachnoid space following the movements of the polytome table. At surgery, a considerable epidural hematoma was removed together with the bullet. (Patient referred for gas myelography from the Department of Neurosurgery, University of Geneva.)

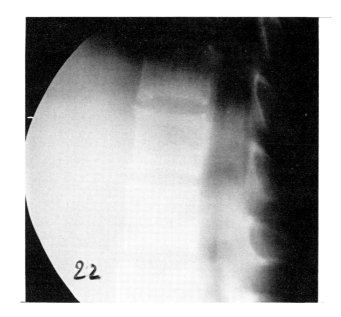

FIGURE 4B

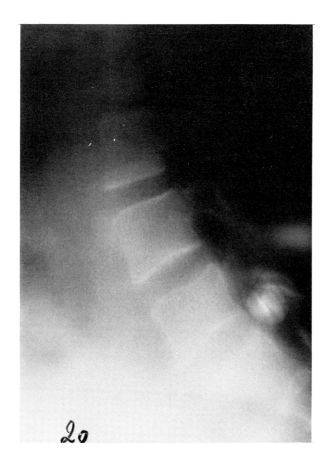

FIGURE 4C

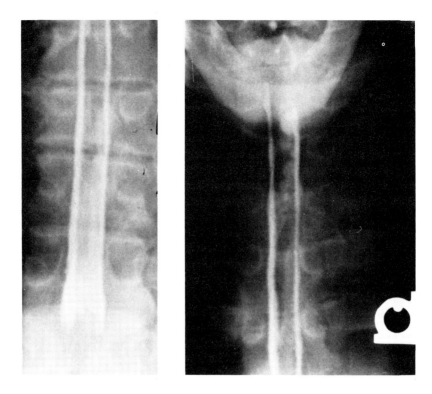

FIGURE 5.   Severe injury to the cervical and thoracic spine was followed by Panto-
paque® myelography. The contrast was injected into the suboccipital area and a complete
block caused by an epidural hematoma was visualized at Th₇. The spinal cord is clearly
outlined between the columns of the opaque medium in the subarachnoid gutters. Edema
of the spinal cord, epidural hematoma, and fracture of vertebrae were found at surgery.

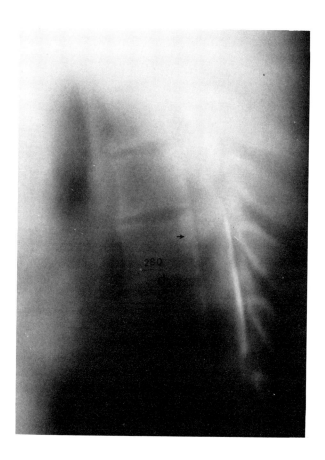

A

FIGURE 6(A). The patient, a 29-year-old male, became paraplegic after falling from a tree. Myelography was performed followed by operation but the patient remained paraplegic. Five years after the accident he was admitted because, in addition to paraplegia, a sensory level developed in the upper left extremity accompanied by back pain. The pain was aggravated and expanded upwards by coughing and straining. Suboccipital instillation of Pantopaque® was carried out first. This myelography disclosed a complete block at Th_{11}. Suboccipital insufflation was done next. The gas myelogram shows a diffusely swollen spinal cord in the thoracic area. Streaks of fixed Pantopaque® are seen dorsally (arrow). (B) The spinal cord is severely compressed at Th_{11} to Th_{12} by the fractured vertebral body. In this area the spinal cord is flattened and atrophic. The subarachnoid space is partially obstructed and the streaks of Pantopaque® are visible (arrows). (C) Gas myelogram demonstrates the compressed and atrophic spinal cord encompassed by oxygen and partly by Pantopaque®. At surgery, thick, extensive meningeal adhesions were separated and the swollen cord was exposed. Multiple cysts, not communicating with the subarachonid space, were found in the spinal cord. This secondary syringomyelia caused by injury associated with spinal cord atrophy and meningeal adhesions was clearly demonstrated by means of gas myelography.

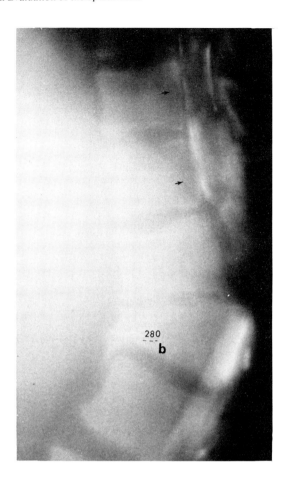

FIGURE 6B

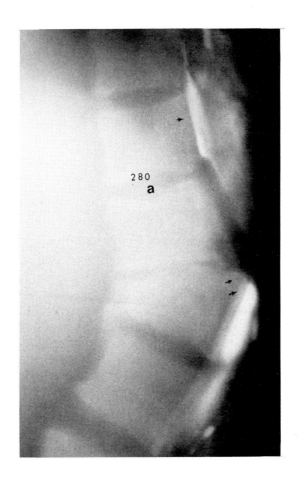

FIGURE 6C

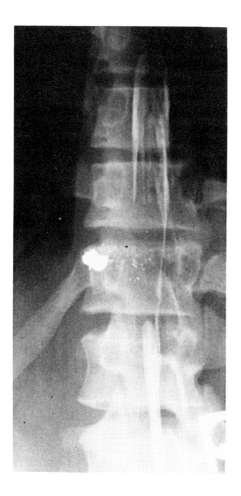
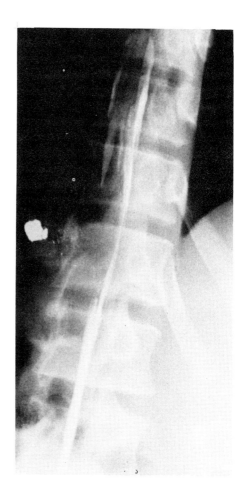

A   B

FIGURE 7.   The patient, male, 25 years old, received a bullet wound followed by paraplegia. Lumbar puncture showed fresh blood in the CSF. (A) Pantopaque® myelogram in the prone shows the bullet that entered the spinal canal from the right side, passed through the meninges and spinal cord, and exited from the canal on its left side. Fine metallic fragments are seen at Th_{12}. The spinal cord is diffusely swollen and the meninges torn. The subarachnoid gutter is narrowed. (B) In the oblique projection the swelling of the spinal cord is well delineated extending from Th_{10} to L_1. On the basis of this myelographic study it was concluded that the injury caused intramedullary, subarachnoid, and epidural hematomas. At surgery these conclusions were confirmed including a considerable tear of the meninges.

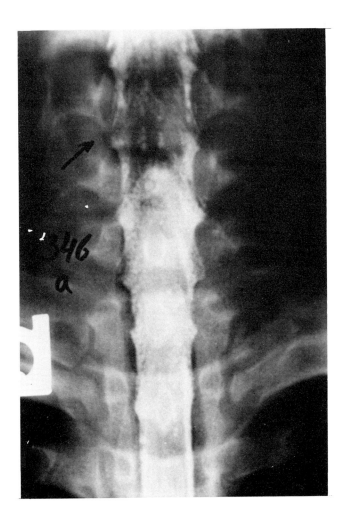

FIGURE 8. The patient, male, 17 years old, sustained a severe neck injury in an automobile accident and developed acute signs of cervical spinal cord compression. Suboccipital myelogram outlines a wide spinal cord between C_3 and C_6 with the contrast medium leakage at C_6. The anterior spinal artery is partially visible. The myelographic finding indicates the presence of posttraumatic spinal cord edema in the cervical region. There is avulsion of a nerve root. At surgery the findings were confirmed.

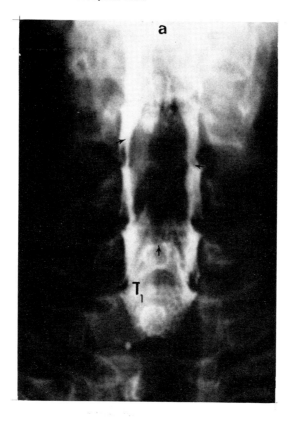

A

FIGURE 9(A).   Pantopaque® myelography was performed following neck injury in this 53-year-old male patient due to the rapidly progressing quadriplegia. In anteroposterior projection, a swollen spinal cord is seen between C_7 and C_4. The nerve roots are wide. The radiolucency of the cord is not homogenous. (B) In moderately oblique positions, the intramedullary lesion is clearly outlined. Considerably enlarged nerve roots are prominent. Small leakage of the contrast medium is seen at C_3 on the left side. The radiologic findings indicated the presence of a posttraumatic intramedullary hemorrhage with nerve root edema and avulsion. These findings were confirmed at surgery. The hematoma in the spinal cord was more concentrated in one area, which may explain the uneven radiolucency of the affected portion of the spinal cord.

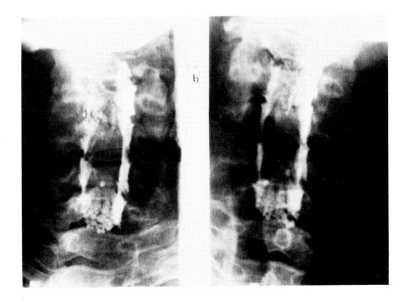

FIGURE 9B

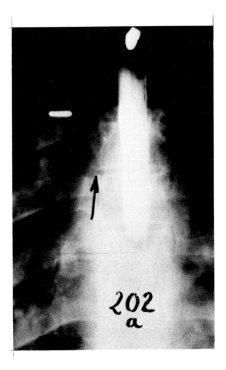

A

FIGURE 10.   The patient, male, 27 years old, received a bullet wound at Th$_1$. Laminectomy was performed but the bullet was not found. Several months later, the patient developed more prominent signs of spinal cord compression. Pantopaque® myelography was carried out. (A) A complete block of the subarachnoid space was disclosed at Th$_2$. The bullet was seen above the obstructed area moving freely according to the changes of the table positions (B) Suboccipital puncture was done and the contrast medium reached the upper pole of what appeared to be a cyst harboring the bullet. At second surgery, a rather large cyst was found compressing the spinal cord with the bullet inside its cavity. The bullet was free in the fluid filling the cyst.

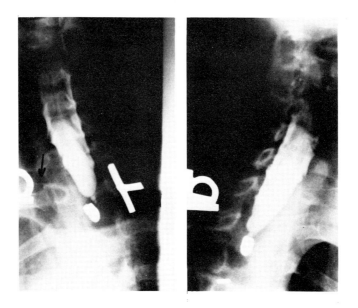

FIGURE 10B

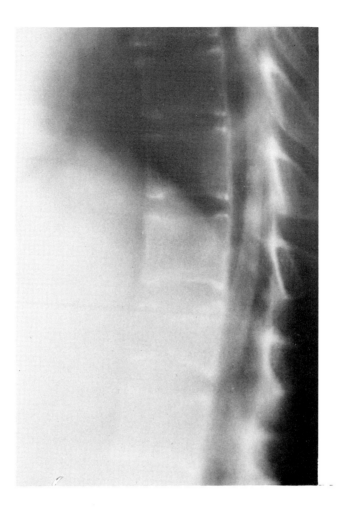

FIGURE 11. Atrophy of the distal end of the spinal cord. Above the atrophic segment the contours of the spinal cord are not demarcated due to adhesions that surround the cord. In the thoracic area the spinal cord is fixed to the dorsal wall of the subarachnoid space. The ventral subarachnoid compartment is wide and filled with gas, whereas the posterior one remained unfilled. This 28-year-old male patient had a severe injury to the upper thoracic region with a fracture of Th₃ vertebra. A large epidural hematoma was found at surgery. The patient remained paraplegic. This gas myelography was performed 2 years following the trauma.

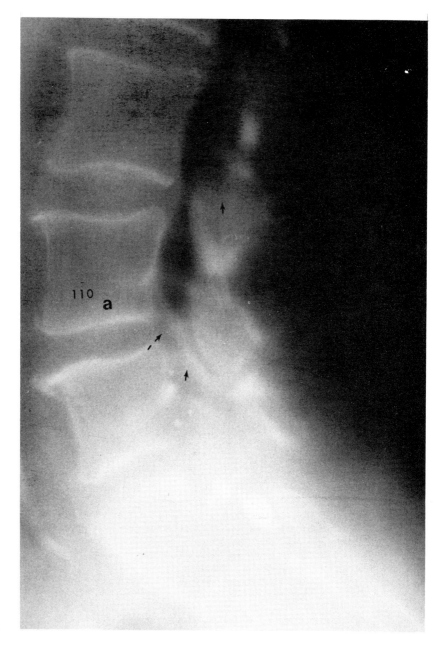

A

FIGURE 12.   This 75-year-old female patient fell off a bicycle and fractured L_1 vertebra. She was admitted three months later because of a persistent back pain. (A) Gas myelography was performed and smaller and larger drops of Pantopaque® were disclosed trapped in the sacral area. Oxygen could not penetrate below L_4 level. The subarachnoid space can be seen as narrow and of an irregular shape. (B) The distal end of the spinal cord is clearly visualized on this gas myelogram showing also small disk protrusions in the upper lumbar region. Above the tip of the needle the subarachnoid space is compressed. At surgery, diffuse adhesions were found in the lumbar region with a larger cyst below L_4 level and a disk herniation at L_4 to L_5. The herniated disk was blocking the canal in this area.

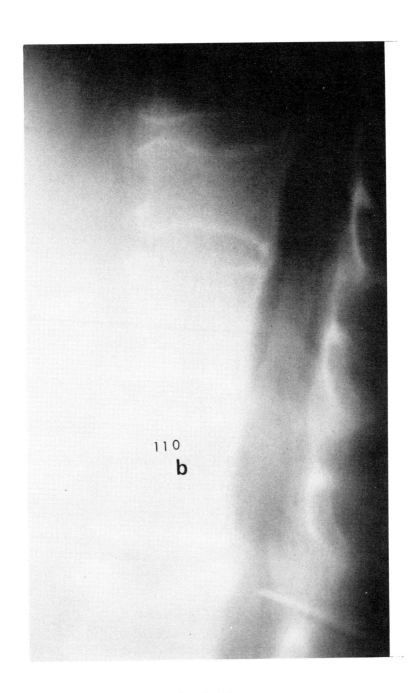

FIGURE 12B

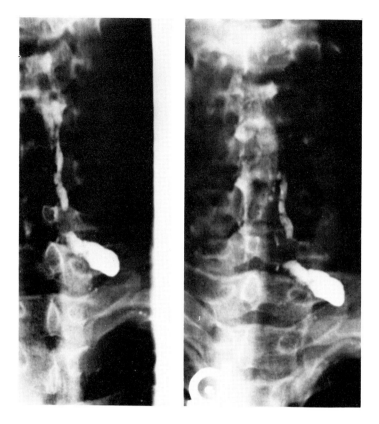

FIGURE 13.   Pantopaque® myelogram reveals the leakage of the contrast medium at C₇ to Th₁ level on the right side, characteristic of a nerve avulsion. The cervical spinal cord is enlarged due to edema and the subarachnoid gutters are almost completely obliterated. The patient, a 30-year-old male, had a severe neck injury in an automobile accident. At surgery, a considerable tear of the meninges and root avulsion were found.

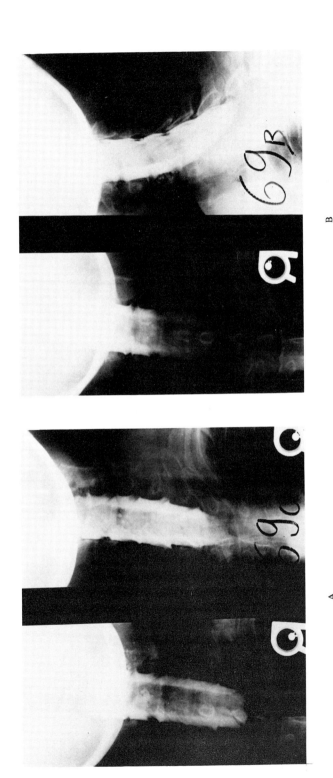

A

B

FIGURE 14. Severe neck injury followed by acute signs of cervical myeloradiculopathy. Myelography with Pantopaque® was performed disclosing the following. (A) In the prone anteroposterior posture, the radiculomedullary arteries reaching the anterior spinal artery are visible in the lower cervical region. A discreet leakage of the contrast medium is seen at C_3 on the right side (arrow). (B) In the oblique position, similar leakage of the contrast medium is discerned at C_4 and C_5 on the left side indicating multiple tears of the dura and nerve root avulsions. The myelographic findings were confirmed at surgery.

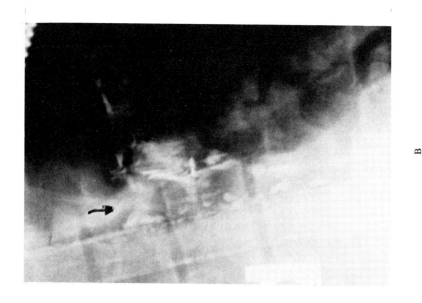

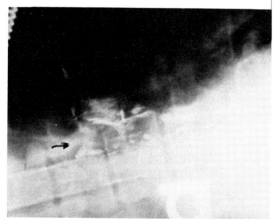

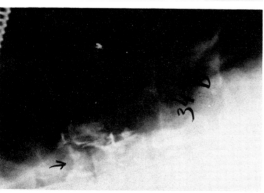

B

A

FIGURE 15.   This 17-year-old female patient was in an automobile accident and fractured the C_5 vertebra. A suboccipital instillation of Pantopaque® was performed. (A) The myelogram of an edema of the spinal cord with nerve root avulsion in the thoracic area. The leakage of the contrast is abundant. (B) A magnified myelogram of the nerve root avulsion. At surgery the radiologic findings were confirmed.

REFERENCES

1. Slager, M., *Basic Neuropathology*, Williams & Wilkins, Baltimore, 1970, chap. 3.
2. Hughes, J. T., *Pathology of the Spinal Cord*, W. B. Saunders, Philadelphia, 1978, chap. 5.
3. Pear, B. L., Spinal epidural hematoma, *Am. J. Roentgenol.*, 115, 155, 1972.
4. Epstein, B. S., *The Spine*, 4th ed., Lea & Febiger, Philadelphia, 1976, 769.
5. Boyd, H. R. and Pear, R. L., Chronic spontaneous spinal epidural hematoma, *J. Neurosurg.*, 36, 239, 1972.
6. Schiller, F., Neligan, G., Budtz-Olsen, O., Surgery in hemophilia — a case of spinal subdural hematoma producing paraplegia, *Lancet*, 2, 842, 1948.
7. Schlang, H. A., Carmichael, A. H., and Freund, C. J., Spontaneous subdural hematoma in anticoagulant therapy, *Am. Pract.*, 13, 247, 1962.
8. Stewart, D. H., Jr. and Watkins, E. S., Spinal cord compression by chronic subdural hematoma. Case report, *J. Neurosurg.*, 31, 80, 1969.
9. Epstein, B. S. and Epstein, J. A., Extrapleural intrathoracic apical traumatic pseudomeningocele, *Am. J. Roentgenol.*, 120, 887, 1974.
10. Nassar, S. I. and Correll, J. W., Subarachnoid hemorrhage due to spinal cord tumors, *Neurology*, 18, 87, 1968.
11. Rinaldi, I. and Peach, W .F., Jr., Postoperative lumbar meningocele, *J. Neurosurg.*, 30, 504, 1969.
12. Pear, B. L., Iatrogenic intraspinal sequestration cysts, *Radiology*, 92, 251, 1969.
13. Rinaldi, I. and Hodges, T. O., Iatrogenic lumbar meningocele: report of three cases, *J. Neurol. Neurosurg. Psychiatry*, 33, 484, 1970.
14. Rossier, A. B., Werner, A., Widi, E., and Berney, J., Contribution to the study of late cervical syringomyelia syndromes after dorsal or lumbar traumatic paraplegia, *J. Neurol. Neurosurg. Psychiatry*, 31, 99, 1968.
15. Bishof, W. and Nittner, K., Zur klinik und Pathogenese der vaskulär bedingten Myelomalazien, *Neurochirugia Stuttg.*, 8, 215, 1965.
16. Barnett, H. J. M., Botterell, E. H., Jousse, A. T., and Wynn-Jones, M., Progressive myelopathy as a sequel to traumatic paraplegia, *Brain*, 89, 159, 1966.
17. Hinkel, C. L. and Nichols, R. L., Opaque myelography in penetrating wounds of the spinal canal, *Am. J. Roentgenol.*, 55, 689, 1946.
18. Heon, M., Myelogram: A questionable aid in diagnosis and prognosis in avulsion of brachial plexus components by traction injuries, *Conn. Med.*, 29, 260, 1965.
19. Alker, G. L., Jr., Glasauer, F. E., Zoll, J. G., and Schagenhauff, R., Myelographic demonstration of lumbosacral nerve root avulsion, *Radiology*, 89, 101, 1967.
20. Harris, W. R., Rathbum, J. B., Wortzman, G., and Humphrey, J. G., Avulsion of lumbar roots complicating fracture of the pelvis, *J. Bone J. Surg.*, 55-A, 1436, 1973.
21. Murphy, F., Hartung, W., and Kirlin, J. W., Myelographic demonstration of avulsion injury of the brachial plexus, *Am. J. Roentgenol.*, 58, 102, 1947.
22. Patterson, F. P. and Morton, K. S., Neurologic complications of fractures and dislocations of the pelvis, *Surg. Gynecol. Obstet.*, 112, 702, 1961.
23. Finney, L. A. and Wulfman, W .A., Traumatic intradural lumbar nerve root avulsion with associated traction injury to common peroneal nerve, *Am. J. Roentgenol.*, 84, 952, 1960.
24. Goodell, C. L., Neurological deficits associated with pelvic fracutres, *J. Neurosurg.*, 24, 837, 1966.
25. Hughes, J. T., Diseases of the spine and spinal cord, in *Greenfield's Neuropathology*, 3rd ed., Blackwood, W. and Corsellis, J. A. N., Eds., Edward Arnold Publication, distributed by Year Book Medical Publishers, Chicago, 1976, 683.
26. Goodman, J. H., Bingham, W. G., Jr., and Hunt, W. E., Platelet aggregation in experimental spinal cord injury, *Arch. Neurol. Chicago*, 36, 197, 1979.

Chapter 10

NEOPLASMS

I. INTRODUCTION

The descriptions related to the tumors of the spinal cord probably came first from Morgagni in 1761, and Phillips in 1792.[1] There were different classifications proposed for the intraspinal tumors, but the one mostly used is based on the cell type, suggested by Bailey and Cushing in 1926.[2] Primary tumors that arise in the spinal cord or surrounding meninges should be differentiated from the secondary invading tumors. According to their location, spinal tumors are classified into two major groups: intramedullary and extramedullary. This topographic differentiation of neoplasms is necessary since their clinical, pathologic, and radiologic features vary depending on their location.[9]

The damage caused to the spinal cord by intramedullary tumors is created through a direct destruction of the normal tissue. The lesion in the cord may be a slowly progressive infiltration or a rapid destruction of the normal tissue caused by a tumor. The damage to the spinal cord in extramedullary neoplasms, on the other hand, is more complex. The basic effect of the tumor on the spinal cord comes as a progressive pressure that affects the normal dynamics of the spinal cord blood circulation. An interference with the venous return, appearing as enlarged serpentine veins below the compression, is usually the first sign of vascular disturbances. Later, the blood circulation can be completely obstructed and arterial pulsations absent. An irreversible damage to the cord will occur if there is a severe compression of nerve fibers and an impaired arterial circulation.[7,50] Tarlov's experimental work suggests that the mechanical pressure is the initial cause of the spinal cord damage, and not the vascular obstruction with a subsequent ischemia. A compression paralysis occurs promptly, whereas the one caused by ischemia takes a longer period of time to develop.[3] This direct pressure interferes with the conduction in the spinal cord and nerve roots. The compression of the ascending longitudinal spinal veins provokes edema of the spinal cord below the site of compression, and the obstruction to the blood flow in the longitudinal and radicular spinal arteries leads to an ischemia of the segments involved. Vascular disturbances that can occur as a result of any pressure to the cord including that caused by tumors, produce edema, degeneration of the ganglion cells and of the white matter, and the development of softening known as compression myelitis. Usually, a gradual spinal compression affects the corticospinal (pyrimidal) tracts first, the posterior columns next, and the spinothalamic tracts last.[4-6,50]

Obstruction to the subarachnoid space prevents the normal flow of the CSF below the point of tumor, thus causing characteristic changes in its composition. The lumbar puncture preceding the instillation of the contrast medium if myelography is carried out, will show xanthochromia with an unusually high content of protein in the spinal fluid. The protein level can be more than 0.5 g/100 mℓ, and a spontaneous coagulation of the CSF may occur, too. In extramedullary tumors, the rise in protein content of the spinal fluid is usually higher than in intramedullary tumors or other space-occupying lesions. Occasionally, the protein content is normal, or slightly raised when the cord is compressed in the cervical region. In tumors of the cauda equina, a high concentration of protein in the spinal fluid has been observed if the fluid is collected above the site of compression.[4,5] The pressure of the fluid below the seat of tumors is subnormal, and the variations in pressure related to the pulse and respiration are often diminished or absent. Queckenstedt's test shows no alterations in the pressure of the fluid below a complete obstruction, and the rise and fall of the pressure may be slower than normal if the obstruction is incomplete. With the patient in the prone position prior to myelography, the abdominal compression, holding of breath, eventual coughing or sneezing may raise the pressure of the CSF even below the obstruction. Hence, the normal Queckenstedt test does not present a certain proof that the spinal compression is absent. As this test is not sufficiently accurate, many investigators have discarded it since myelography can provide more exact information about the state of the spinal canal and cord.[12,14,15] In distally situated tumors, especially in those of the cauda equina, it may be impossible to obtain the CSF by lumbar puncture, in which case a cisternal or lateral cervical puncture should be carried out to obtain the fluid, and the instillation of the contrast medium can be done from above. In the presence of a subarachnoid block caused by a tumor, the lumbar puncture associated with the collection of the CSF below the level of obstruction may cause a shift in the position of the tumor, which further on may lead to temporary or even permanent intensification of the symptoms, especially root pain, weakness, and retention of urine.[4,5,7] In case of a suspected spinal tumor, lumbar puncture and myelography should be carried out cautiously, and it is advisable to discuss with the attending neurosurgeon the possibility of operating immediately if such aggravation of the symptoms should occur following myelography.

Clinical signs in spinal tumors usually develop in a gradual fashion; however, a rapid onset of carcinoma of the vertebral column and of an acute compression is possible. About two thirds of the patients who develop spinal tumors undergo surgery between the 1st and 2nd year follwoing the appearance of initial clinical signs.[4,5] Sometimes, this interval can be longer. Initial symptoms in spinal cord tumors are usually sensory, manifested as a radiating pain in the distrubution of one or more spinal nerves. The pain becomes more accentuated if the tumor has an extramedullary location, especially in case of a neurofibroma. Root pain is less pronounced in intramedullary tumors. The pain, either unilateral or bilateral, is often described as a constricting or burning sensation, commonly associated with tenderness of the skin or deeper tissues. Movements of the spine, coughing, or sneezing may intensify the sensation of the pain. The back pain is particularly frequent in tumors of the cauda equina. Tumors of the cervical spine may provoke an unpleasant distant pain in the lower limbs since there is an involvement of the spinothalamic tracts. In most instances, motor symptoms develop later than the sensory. Therefore, stiffness, unsteadiness, or weakness of the extremities will follow. In compression of the cervical spinal cord, motor symptoms involve first one upper limb, then the lower extremity on the same side followed by the opposite lower limb, and finally the opposite upper limb.[4,19] If the compression is localized below the cervical enlargement of the spinal cord, motor signs are limited to the lower limbs only. A rapid development of paraplegia is unusual in tumors but quite common in extension or flexion injuries of the neck. The disturbances of the sphincters often appear later, even if the tumor involves the conus or cauda equina.[8,19]

Progressive weakness, wasting, and fasciculations of the muscles are present in case of compression of ventral roots, or of the anterior horns of the grey matter. Spastic weakness of the muscles below the level of the tumor will be found in case of corticospinal tract compression. The compression of the dorsal spinal roots can further on cause hyperesthesia and hyperalgesia in the affected cutaneous segments. Anesthesia and analgesia may develop later. Flexion and extension of the cervical spine, if the spinal cord is compressed, frequently cause pain, numbness, or tingling radiating into the area innervated by the segment of the spinal cord affected by the lesion. This symptom (Lhermitte's sign) may be provoked by both intramedullary and extramedullary tumors, and should be taken into consideration in the process of positioning the patient for the myelographic study.[4,19,50]

Spinal tumors call for a careful evaluation of standard radiographs prior to any further radiologic examination. Radiographs of the spine are often combined with tomography and their evaluation is important because it allows, in many instances, the exclusion of the presence of different lesions such as fractures that may compress the spinal cord and meninges and produce symptoms similar to those caused by a tumor. In addition, standard radiographs will demonstrate, in about 15 to 20% of cases, changes caused by a spinal tumor. The common findings are an enlargement of the spinal canal, presence of calcifications that may be discreet and difficult to recognize, enlargement of intervertebral foramen because of the protrusion of the neoplasm, and changes of the contours of the spine and paravertebral tissue. Metastatic tumors involving the bony structures of the spine often affect, through expansion or compression, the spaces and tissues of the spinal canal. On the other hand, the spinal cord tumors usually do not invade the bony structures, and they do not give metastases outside the nervous system.[12,14,15,37,39]

II. INTRAMEDULLARY TUMORS

Intramedullary tumors have been the subject of many experimental and clinical studies. A number of statistics show that the most common intramedullary tumors are *ependymomas* and *astrocytomas*.[7,50] The statistics done by Sloof and co-workers indicate that there is a certain difference in the types of tumors involving the spinal cord and brain.[5,6] The incident of intramedullary tumors in adults varies from 7 to 22%.[5-7] Approximately 22.5% of all intraspinal tumors are intramedullary *gliomas*.[8] This presents a considerable difference in comparision with brain tumors where gliomas constitute over 50% of all primary intracranial neoplasms. In adults, the spinal cord neoplasms are mostly located in the thoracic region.[9] Considering all intraspinal tumors, their occurrence in children is more frequent in the cervical, lumbar, and sacral regions, probably due to the frequency of congenital anomalies in these areas.[10,11,13] Equally, gliomas and different types of congenital tumors are more commonly seen in children. Extramedullary and intradural tumors, however, are present more often in adults than in children.[6,11-13]

In intramedullary tumors, myelography provides a higher diagnostic accuracy than any other radiologic procedure. Prior to myelography, it is advantageous to carefully evaluate the clinical symptomatology and the general state of the patient. Myelography in intramedullary tumors should be carefully planned and well executed. It is advisable to appraise the appearance of the spinal fluid and collect a minimal amount needed for laboratory tests. The contrast medium, opaque or lucent, is usually injected in the lumbar area. However, if an extensive tumor blocks the lumbar region, it may be necessary to carry out the instillation of the contrast medium in the lateral cervical or suboccipital area. On some occasions, there may be a need to outline the upper pole of the tumor, for which reason the contrast medium is injected in the suboccipital or cervical subarachnoid space. Most commonly, a small amount of opaque, insoluble contrast media is used in the presence of a subarachnoid block. Opinions differ as to the quantity of the contrast agent used in the presence of a tumor of the spinal cord.[14,15,43] In case of a complete obstruction of the subarachnoid space, mostly about 4 cc of the contrast agent is sufficient to outline the lower pole of the tumor. If the contrast medium can bypass the intramedullary neoplasm in the narrowed subarachnoid gutter, a few more cubic centimeters can be added in order to achieve a satisfactory delineation of the tumor's contour. Often, gas can encompass the intramedullary expansive lesion more completely than insoluble contrast media. Equally, Metrizamide® may bypass the obstruction and outline the surface of the swollen cord, and provide more information about the neoplasm. The fusiform expansion or spindle-like configuration of the spinal cord, demonstrated by myelography, is not pathognomonic for an invasive intramedullary tumor. A number of different pathologic lesions, such as edema of different origin, can present a similar picture. It is necessary to evaluate the lesion by means of fluoroscopy and spot radiography, in all projections, to obtain the optimal information. At times, it is possible to pass insoluble contrast media beyond the obstruction and outline the upper margin of the tumor if the patient is kept for several minutes in a head-down position. The deformity of the cord caused by a tumor is greatest at the level of the center of the lesion. The width of the cord gradually diminishes in the caudal and cranial directions to merge with the normal spinal cord. The arachnoid gutters on both sides of the cord are narrowed, particularly at the level of the central part of the lesion. The enlarged segment of the cord that can be identified by means of myelography does not necessarily represent the size of the tumor since the associated edema or hemorrhage may contribute to the deformity of the cord, and the spreading of the tumor can be present in the apparently normal parts of the spinal cord.[7,50] Neoplasm can infiltrate the tissue of the spinal cord over a number of segments before the level of obstruction is encountered. At the level of maximal obstruction, the contrast medium, diverted upward, encircles the expanded mass in narrow streaks or droplets. The streak of an opaque contrast medium can extend over several segments. The contrast agent usually fills the arachnoid sleeves surrounding the nerve roots, giving a beaded appearance to the subarachnoid space. The unimpeded visualization of the nerve sleeves is rather characteristic of an intramedullary tumor, whereas extramedullary neoplasms mostly obstruct the nerve root pouches. Below the obstructed area, distended and tortuous venous channels may be demonstrated around the swollen cord.[12,14,18,23,39]

Intramedullary tumors arising from individual nerve roots of the cauda equina often cannot be distinguished from any other intradural lesion. Gliomas of the nerve can expand and obliterate the subarachnoid space forming a smooth obstruction to the flow of the contrast medium. These tumors can often be outlined if gas or Metrizamide® is used. Some of these gliomas will sometimes have an irregular shape and expand along the nerve roots. The eccentric gulf of the tumor in the spinal cord is rare, particularly in comparison with tumors of the cauda equina.[9,14,15]

The enlargement of the spinal cord resulting from the growth of an intramedullary neoplasm is ordinarily shorter than the enlargement seen in syringomyelia where the dilatation may involve many segments of the cord. Yet the length of the enlargement cannot be considered as a reliable differential diagnostic criterion because, occasionally, ependymoma or astrocytoma will infiltrate a considerable length of the spinal cord.[5-7]

Ependymoma is a slow-growing tumor arising from the ependymal lining of the central canal. It occurs either in the spinal cord or in the filum terminale. Ependymoma comprises about 60 to 70% of intramedullary tumors and it appears slightly more often in males, usually between 32 and 40 years, and somewhat earlier in females.[7,24,50] This tumor is inclined towards slow growth, and it is mostly situated in the caudal part of the cord, and especially in the filum terminale. Usually, it is soft and well demarcated from the surrounding spinal cord tissue and may appear with a pseudo capsule. Ependymoma of the filum terminale is commonly free among the nerves that form the cauda equina, and has the characteristics of benign tumors. However, it may assume an infiltrative growth involving meninges, nerve roots, and even bone. Some investigators have observed that ependymoma and some other spinal cord tumors can be associated with syringomyelia. It should be mentioned though, that small cyst formations found in ependymomas cannot be associated with syringomyelia.[8] Ependymoma may be of a considerable size, and may extend along the filum terminale filling the subarachnoid space. Ependymoma of a large size has been known as a giant tumor of the cauda equina.[14,15,34] Myelography will occasionally show a tongue-like extension of the tumor within the lumbar subarachnoid space. This feature may help differentiate this type of tumor from other gliomas. Sometimes, ependymoma will displace the cord and cause a relative or complete block of the subarachnoid space. If the growth of the tumor is symmetrical in the spinal cord, a widening of the cord occurs, and the obstruction of the subarachnoid space demonstrated by means of myelography will not be characteristic of ependymoma* (Figure 1).[8,14,15,39]

Astrocytoma of the spinal cord represents, according to the statistics of Sloof and co-workers, 3.05% of all astrocytomas of the CNS, which approximately corresponds to the weight of the spinal cord being 2.57% of the total weight of the nervous tissue.[5] Astrocytomas tend to spring up in all parts of the spinal cord. This tumorous infiltration of the cord may be quite extensive. It appears somewhat more often in males than in females. It is found in children or elderly people, and it occurs between 3 and 73 years. Astrocytoma often produces a fusiform expansion of the spinal cord that may obliterate completely the subarachnoid space. The tumor is usually firm. Within an astrocytoma, cystic degeneration is common. Cavitations may look as if simulating syringomyelia.[6,11] Different microscopic types of astrocytomas grading from 1 to 4 can be encountered in the spinal cord.[6,7] For example, the more slowly growing grade 1 astrocytoma is the dominant tumor of this type. The grade 4, on the other hand, is rare in the spinal cord. Astrocytomas represent about 30% of intramedullary gliomas. A widening of the cord is a common myelographic finding in astrocytomas with possible bony erosions and scoliosis of the dorsal spine. Filling the subarachnoid space with oxygen may help outline the upper and lower poles of the tumor and its margins. In other instances, an uncharacteristic block of the subarachnoid space can be demonstrated by means of myelography. Eventually, a contrast medium in this situation could be injected into the cervical or suboccipital subarachnoid space so that the outlining of the upper pole of the tumor becomes visible (Figures 2 and 3).[4,5,11,23,24]

Oligodendroglioma is a rare, slow growing, and often encapsulated tumor of the spinal cord. If removed, the prognosis of the patient is mostly good. Ganglioma, neuroblastoma, and ganglioneuroma are rare tumors of the spinal cord, benign in nature, and very slow growing. Although a primary neuroblastoma of the spinal cord is infrequent, the dissemination of the cerebellar medulloblastoma into the spinal cord is quite common.[5,6]

Teratoma is a neoplasm composed of different tissues with no resemblance to the spinal cord. Teratoma in the spinal cord is also quite rare, yet if it occurs, it is mostly localized in the cervical and lumbosacral regions, and it is often associated with different developmental abnormalities, such as spina bifida.[16] The inner part of the tumor usually consists of a cyst containing a fluid of mucinous or caseous nature. Microscopic analyses of a teratoma reveal various types of tissues of ectodermal or mesodermal origin. The presence of embryonal tissue often determines the malignancy of a teratoma. Myelographic findings in the presence of this type of tumor are not characteristic.[13,37,41,50]

Dermoid and epidermoid cysts in the spinal cord occur somewhat more often than teratomas, and there have been several good reports concerning these types of developmental cysts.[5-7,47] They are found at any level of the spinal cord, but more often in the distal part. These cysts can have an intramedullary or extramedullary location, or they may appear partially inside and partially outside the spinal cord. In a typical

---

* All figures appear following the text.

fashion, they represent an expanding mass of the cauda equina, often so large that it can completely fill the subarachnoid space. Widening of the interpedicular space, or erosions of the pedicles and posterior surface of the vertebral bodies associated with developmental abnormalities, such as spina bifida, are common in these types of cysts. Myelographic findings are not characteristic and vary depending upon the location and extension of the cysts. In most instances, a complete block of the subarachonid space is seen on myelograms.

Lipoma is equally an infrequent intramedullary tumor, often associated with bony anomalies, especially with spina bifida.[17] This tumor, made out of adult fat cells, is difficult to differentiate on myelographic studies from other intramedullary neoplasms. In three of our cases of lipomas, Pantopaque® myelography showed the widening of the spinal cord. The narrow streaks of the contrast medium were diverging in the compressed subarachnoid gutters encircling the lower pole of the enlarged spinal cord in the shape of the letter V (Figure 4). The tendency of the contrast medium to bypass the obstruction suggested that the tumor within the spinal cord could be of an elastic and soft consistency. On surgery, the tumor had a rather extensive growth involving several segments of the spinal cord. Lipomas were the subject of a number of reviews because of their infrequent intramedullary occurrence.[7,17,41,50]

Hemangioblastoma is a seldom occurring, well vascularized tumor of the spinal cord.[5,18] On several occasions, we reported cases of intramedullary hemangioblastomas observed on myelograms and sometimes on angiograms of the spinal cord. More recently, we have described radiologic features in correlation with surgical and pathologic findings related to this type of tumor. In the series of 18 spinal cord hemangioblastomas, three had an abrupt onset and neurological signs of cervical cord compression due to the hemorrhage. In the remaining 15 patients, the symptoms of the spinal cord compression, on the average, progressed to plegia in 2 years. In six patients, the spinal cord hemangioblastomas were related to the von Hippel-Lindeau complex transmitted as a dominant trait. A family history of retinal and cerebellar tumors could be traced only in one of the six patients. The median age of the 18 patients at the onset of the spinal cord symptoms was 34 years. In two patients, vascularized associated tumors were present, one in the pancreas and the other in the kidneys. On myelography, the widening of the spinal cord with pronounced tortuous venous channels was found in most of these tumors (Figures 5 and 6). The angiography showed vascularized, single, or multiple lesions.[20,45]

Some exceptionally rare tumors such as malignant fibrosarcoma of the filum terminale and the intramedullary schwannomas can affect the spinal cord.[50] Equally rare are metastatic tumors of the spinal cord.[35] Bronchogenic carcinoma appears to be the most frequent origin of metastases in the spinal cord, whereas the metastases of a breast carcinoma, kidney carcinoma, malignant melanoma, and adrenal carcinoma are less common.[21,22,29,33] On a post-mortem study, Chason and co-workers found metastatic lesions in the spinal cord in 1% of all cases of carcinoma, including malignant melanoma.[22] Clinical signs of a malignant secondary invasion of the spinal cord may not be evident at all times due to the general status of the patients. Metastatic tumors of the spinal cord originating from the brain, however, seem to be more frequent.[14,35] The dissemination of the tumors occurs probably through the circulation of the spinal fluid. The most common tumors of the brain that can give metastases to the spinal cord are glioblastoma multiforme, medulloblastoma, pinealoma, epndymoma, and hemangioblastoma. This type of metastasis may take place at any level of the spinal cord, and may be multiple. A complete or partial obstruction of the subarachnoid space or multiple defects will show on myelograms without radiographic signs of destruction of the bony structures. Metastases can also invade the region of the cauda equina and cause a displacement of the nerves.[7,50]

It should be noted that the primary tumors of the spinal cord are infrequent in the newborn, and if they occur, they are usually developmental neoplasms such as teratomas, lipomas, dermoids, or neurenteric cysts.[50] Exceptionally rare neuroblastoma and primary glioma of the spinal cord have been reported in literature. Equally infrequent are the tumors originating from supporting vascular and connective tissue of the spinal cord. Recently, a case of meningeal sarcoma of the spinal cord has been described in a newborn.[51]

III. EXTRAMEDULLARY TUMORS OF THE SPINE

Extramedullary tumors of the spine can be divided into two major groups: intradural and extradural neoplasms. Extramedullary intradural tumors comprise about 50 to 65% of all tumors of the spine and the extradural about 25 to 30%. Some of these tumors, approximately 11%, can be both intradural and extradural.[9,23,24] The damage to the spinal cord inflicted by these neoplasms will depend to a great extent upon their growth. If it is a slow growing neoplasm, benign in nature, the spinal cord will be gradually compressed. If, however, it is a malignant infiltrative and destructive type of tumor, either primary or secondary in origin, the spinal cord will be invaded by the tumor tissue. The two most common benign tumors affecting the spinal canal and cord are neurofibroma and meningioma.

Neurofibroma and schwannoma have spurred some discussions concerning their nomenclature.[6] Neurofibromas are often multiple tumors originating from the spinal and cranial nerve roots and from the peripheral nerves. Neurofibroma may look like an expansion of the nerve from which it originates and the nerve appears to transverse the tumor. Schwannoma is usually a solitary tumor, although multiple neoplasms of this type are not uncommon. Schwannoma is encapsulated and appears to be adherent to the nerve rather than transversed by it. Both neurofibroma and schwannoma can affect any of the spinal nerve roots, and they are more mobile than meningeomas since they are not attached to the meninges in most instances. On histologic grounds, schwannomas derive from the neurilemma cells or the sheath of Schwann. Neurofibromas are believed today to be also of Schwannian origin.[6,25] Occasionally, these neoplasms may originate from a nerve root within an intervertebral foramen and extend into the spinal canal and out of the foramen into the thoracic cavity. These tumors are often referred to as "dumbbell tumors" because of their shape.[36,39,40,46]

Neurofibroma (neurolemmoma) and schwannoma occur mostly earlier in life and affect almost equally females and males. Most of them are localized in the thoracic region (43%) and less frequently in the lumbar (33.5%) and cervical (22%).[9,15,25] Some of these benign tumors undergo malignant changes occurring in about 10 to 16% of cases.[23,25] Frequently, benign nerve tumors have an hourglass shape, usually smooth and soft, arising mostly from the posterior nerve roots.

Clinical signs and symptoms linked to the presence of neurofibroma and schwannoma are mainly those of compression of the spinal cord and nerve roots. On radiographs, changes of the bony structures of the spinal canal can be seen in hourglass tumors, however, they are not characteristic and can occur with other types of expanding lesions. Commonly, atrophy of the pedicles, widening of the intervertebral foramina, deformity of the laminae, and erosion of concavity of the posterior surface of the vertebral body will develop in conjunction with these tumors and can be demonstrated on radiographs. Calcifications in neurofibromas and schwannomas are not common. Myelography, either with positive or negative contrast media, will usually disclose a partial or complete block of the subarachnoid space. The spinal cord is in most cases displaced to the opposite side of the tumor and compressed against the wall of the spinal canal (Figure 7). Typically, the filling defect around the tumor is smooth and the convexity of the neoplasm clearly demarcated. Often, it is possible to encompass with the contrast medium, a larger portion of its contour due to the fact that the tumor is not attached to the meninges. Nevertheless, myelographic findings are not pathognomonic and it may prove difficult to distinguish a neurofibroma from a meningioma. Neurofibroma involving one nerve of the cauda equina can be demonstrated on myelograms as a clearly circumscribed tumor (Figure 8). By utilizing gas and water-soluble contrast media, this type of tumor can be clearly delineated and the diagnosis achieved with accuracy. The nerve sheath tumors in the area of cauda equina become quite large, known as "giant tumors", similar to ependymomas. In a dumbbell neurofibroma, a rounded soft tissue is often seen in the paravertebral region associated with enlarged intervertebral foramen and the widening of the spinal canal. The extradural component of the tumor may be considerably larger than the one in the vertebral canal.[14,25,36,37]

Neurofibroma and schwannoma on positive contrast myelography can produce a cup-like accumulation of the contrast medium. The upper margin of this cup-like formation is usually concave upward due to the arrest of the contrast medium at the lower pole of the tumor. Similar configuration of the contrast medium can be seen in meningiomas, too. It is important to demonstrate the tumor in all myelographic projections, and occasionally, it may be necessary to turn the patient supine (Figure 9).[46] The displacement of the spinal cord, as mentioned above, is a characteristic feature of extramedullary subdural space-occupying lesions. A displacement of the spinal cord is rather unusual to see in intramedullary expanding lesions. The intramedullary space-occupying lesions create a diffuse enlargement of the spinal cord, and in case of extramedullary tumors, the spinal cord can be narrowed and rather thin. Ordinarily, a dorsally placed neurofibroma or schwannoma can be detected more accurately by means of gas myelography. This applies, in particular, to the tumors in the area of the foramen magnum and upper cervical region, which should be distinguished from the Arnold-Chiari malformation.

In neurofibromatosis, multiple smaller or larger tumors are distributed around the spinal cord and attached to the nerve roots. Often, they are clustered forming grape-like configurations, and can be clearly demonstrated by means of gas myelography. Seen on gas myelograms, most of the time the spinal cord does not appear displaced, but it may be compressed between the smaller and larger tumors. The spinal canal is not usually enlarged in neurofibromatosis, yet a widening of the subarachnoid space may be found (dural ectasia).[14] The occurrence of neurofibroma with gliosis was described in literature, as well as the thickening of the spinal cord in the thoracic and cervical regions caused by intramedullary neurofibroma.[23] Neurofibromatosis can be associated with hemangioma, or with various developmental abnormalities, and it may constitute the von Recklinghausen disease. Different tumors, such as optic glioma, intracerebral glioma, ganglioneuroma, astrocytoma, and other types of neoplasms can accompany the von Recklinghausen disease.[50]

Meningioma occurs in about 85% of cases in women in middle life. They are localized in approximately 82% in the thoracic area, in 16.5% in the cervical, and in 1.5% in the lumbar region.[6,9,25,50] Meningiomas are, in most instances, attached to the inner surface of the dura and invested by the arachnoid. They are firm, encapsulated, benign tumors that may be adherent to the pia without infiltrating the spinal cord. Rarely, they will have an extradural location and expand into the thorax through an intervertebral foramen appearing with the features of a dumbbell tumor.[26,27] The slow growing psammomatous type of meningioma with abundant calcified concretions is more common in the spinal canal than in intracranial areas. The calcifications within a meningioma of this type can be recognized on standard radiographs in about 4% of cases.[14,15]

Spreading of an intracranial meningioma into the spinal canal, often known as meningioma en-plaque, can be seen occasionally, mostly in younger subjects (Figure 10).
Postoperative recurrence of meningioma is not common.

Clinical signs produced by meningiomas are mainly those of compression of the
spinal cord and nerve roots. However, a meningioma of the rim of the foramen magnum can often expand into the spinal canal (Figure 11). On the other hand, a meningioma pertaining to the upper cervical region will extend into the posterior fossa (Figure 12). This type of meningioma appears with clinical signs related to this particular
area. Frequently, the compression of the spinal cord in the cervico-occipital region is
associated with pain in the proximal segment of the neck, paresthesia, weakness of the
upper limbs, atrophy of the small muscles of the hand, disturbances of the position
sense, and eventually spastic paraparesis. Involvement of the upper spinal and cranial
nerves may occur.

Myelography can demonstrate a partial block of the subarachnoid space with the
visualization of the tumor pole, and the displacement of the spinal cord is more apparent in meningiomas than in neurofibromas. Meningiomas sometimes have a bilobulated surface (Figure 13). They have clear myelographic characteristics of extramedullary and intradural tumors, as described with neurofibromas. If a meningioma is in a
lateral position to the spinal cord, the cup-like defect will be apparent on myelograms.
If, on the other hand, the tumor is located in the midline of the subarachnoid dorsal
or ventral compartment, it will produce a fusiform widening of the spinal cord similar
to the one seen in intramedullary tumors. However, myelograms in the lateral, prone,
or supine position, can demonstrate the extramedullary location of the tumor and the
dorsal or ventral displacement of the spinal cord. The visualization of the tumor in
different projections is essential. A compressed spinal cord can be considerably thinned
by the hard tumor mass in a similar way as in neurofibromas (Figures 14 and 15). If a
meningioma is located distally to the spinal cord, it will cause a displacement of the
nerves of the cauda equina. Occasionally, these tumors can be quite large and difficult
to distinguish from other expansive lesions involving the lumbar area of the spinal
canal (Figure 16). In the region of the foramen magnum, meningiomas are commonly
ventrally placed, however, they do occur in the dorsal area as well (Figure 17). As
mentioned before, tumors in this region should be differentiated from other pathologic
conditions, especially from the Arnold-Chiari malformation. The exploration of this
area by means of gas myelography is more advantageous.[11,12,14,15,25,39]

Meningiomas with neurofibroma and schwannoma comprise approximately 60 to
70% of extramedullary intradural tumors.[7,9,15] Other forms of benign tumors of the
spinal canal are rare. It is uncommon that a cavernous hemangioma of the vertebrae
is the cause of a spinal cord compression (Figure 18). Compression of the spinal cord
occurs rarely in osteoblastoma (osteoid fibroma), osteoclastoma, and osteoid osteoma.
Lipoma has already been described as an intramedullary neoplasm, but it occurs more
frequently as an extramedullary tumor, eventually compressing the spinal cord. Lipoma often has a dorsal position and represents a slowly growing tumor. It is mostly
extradural, but at times it can have an extramedullary and intradural location. Lipoma
appears in younger subjects, and extends over several vertebral segments causing a
widening of the vertebral canal that can be seen on radiographs of the spine. Myelography can demonstrate a partial or complete obstruction of the subarachnoid space
with the characteristics of extramedullary intradural or extradural tumors.[17,37,44,50]

Chordoma is a malignant tumor that arises from the primitive notochord and may
be found at any level of the spine. It is described here together with benign tumors
because of its slow growth and the bony changes that may be similar to those seen in
neurofibroma or meningioma. Chordoma invades the spine locally and is prone to
recurrence. The metastasis originating from chordoma occurs in less than 10% of

cases. Approximately 88% of chordomas are located in the sacrococcygeal region and at the base of the skull. Less commonly, they will have an intraspinal location (12%), mostly extradural, and often in the cervical area.[7,9,50] Chordoma is initially an encapsulated tumor that involves the spinal cord and nerves. Dense calcifications of amorphous shape are often seen within the tumor. The destruction of the vertebral body is usually disclosed first, followed by the invasion of the arch. The involvement of the bone begins early with the appearance of a slowly growing paravertebral mass directed laterally, or located anteriorly to the involved segments of the spine.[28] Chordoma in the region of the clivus may extend towards the spinal canal (Figure 19). The spinal cord and pons may be compressed and displaced posteriorly (Figure 19). On myelograms, the lower pole of the tumor appears delineated, and the subarachnoid space is partially or completely obstructed (Figure 19). A certain degree of spinal cord atrophy due to a long-lasting compression can be detected.[28] Angiography may be combined with myelography in order to localize and estimate the extent of the tumor in the cervico-occipital region (Figure 19). Myelography in chordoma is also used for the postoperative evaluation of the spinal canal for its demonstration following radiation therapy, and in case of recurrence of the tumor.[6,14,23]

Extradural tumors that affect the spinal cord originate from different tissues. Extradural tumors comprise about 30% of all spinal tumors, and the majority are malignant.[7,50] The most common type are metastases of various carcinomas. Metastases involving the spine derive from bronchogenic carcinoma, breast carcinoma, lymphoma, renal carcinoma, myeloma, sarcoma, prostatic carcinoma, rectal carcinoma, uterine carcinoma, and thyroid carcinoma.[29] To these tumors, causing metastatic lesions that may involve the spinal cord, should be added a less common type, such as hepatoma, ovarian carcinoma, seminoma, pancreatic carcinoma, malignant melanoma, and lymphoepithelioma. Occasionally, neuroblastoma and hemangioendothelioma will produce metastases to the spine, too.[7] The primary melanoma of the leptomeninges is a rare neoplasm that has a tendency to expand in a disseminated fashion forming multiple growths.[33] Sporadically, a ganglioneuroma may spread into the spinal canal through an intervertebral foramen.

In case of metastatic and primary extradural tumors, the spinal cord and the nerve roots may be involved in different ways.[29] Paraplegia that occurs as a result of the spinal cord compression may come from a vertebral collapse. If the vertebral bodies are the seat of a primary malignant neoplasm or metastases, the bone destruction may cause a collapse of one or more vertebrae. The collapse can develop rapidly, causing an angulation of the spinal canal (Figure 20). The damage produced to the spinal cord is similar to the one seen in Pott's paraplegia or in osteoporosis. In addition to the purely mechanical effect of the collapsed bony spine on the cord, the malignant infiltration of the spinal canal may be present, too. This type of invasion of the spinal cord and nerve roots is seen particularly in malignant tumors originating from the reticulo-endothelial system.[7,29,35,38] Furthermore, due to an extensive compression caused by extradural tumors, the blood supply to the spinal cord can be impaired. If a neoplasm is surrounding the spinal column, obliteration of radicular tributaries may occur in the intervertebral foramina, and the infarction of a segment of the spinal cord will be the result.

Primary extradural tumors originate from the dura or nerve roots, extradural soft tissues, and vertebrae. Benign extradural tumors comprise meningiomas that may undergo a malignant degeneration, neurofibromas, lipomas, dermoids or epidermoids, and some vascular lesions.[7,50] Tumors of lymphatic origin are the most common primary malignant epidural tumors. Signs of spinal cord or nerve root involvement are the first symptoms in about 5% of patients with Hodgkin's disease, lymphosarcoma, and leukemia. Sarcomas deriving from other than lymphatic tissues in the vertebral canal are uncommon.[51] An epidural sarcoma can generate a soft tissue mass extending into the paravertebral region.[27,30,31] Sarcomas represent about 11% of all primary neoplasms, and they occur more often in the dorsal area. In about 33% of these tumors, the changes on the bones may be seen on radiographs, such as erosion of vertebral body, pedicles, and intervertebral foramina.[14,31] Chondrosarcoma can develop from a benign osteochondroma. Myeloma, tumor of myeloerythropoietic tissue, may arise from the epidural space, and it may involve the spinal canal thus causing the spinal cord compression.[7,31,32] Usually, the dura shows a resistance to the invasion by a myeloma, and its intradural location is rare. Punched out areas of bony destruction can be seen in the region of the spine. The fracture of the spine may not be detectable on radiographs, but later, it can become evident through a proliferation of the bone tissue. Paravertebral soft tissue mass is seen more often on radiographs in myeloma than in metastatic carcinoma. Clinical manifestations in myeloma and lymphoma are related to the compression of the spinal cord (Figure 21).[32] Pain, local or radiating in nature, paresthesia, weakness of the extremities, paraplegia, sensory level disturbances, changes in deep tendon reflexes, and bowel and bladder disturbances, all can be encountered. Many of these clinical signs are not specific for this type of tumor, and they represent general signs of spinal cord involvement. More characteristic are laboratory findings such as anemia, the presence of Bence-Jones protein in urine, hyperproteinemia due to increased globuline fraction. These findings combined with radiographic bony changes can indicate the nature of the tumor (Figure 20).

Metastases of primary malignant tumors affecting the spine produce osteolytic or osteoblastic changes recognizable in about 50 to 60% of cases on standard radiographs and tomograms.[14,39] It should be mentioned, nonetheless, that an extensive involvement of the bony structures of the spine produced by different types of the above-mentioned metastases, may exist without causing changes visible on radiographs. Tumors belonging to the lymphoma type will show on radiographs, in addition to paraspinal soft tissue masses, changes of the bones of osteolytic or osteoblastic character in about 20% of cases.[14,50] Metastases of carcinoma expanding in the extradural space represent extensions from an involved bony component (Figure 22). This is particularly true of breast carcinoma metastases that cause osteolytic, osteoblastic, and often mixed changes of the bony components of the spine. Pathologic fractures are associated with the destruction of the bony elements of the spine in most cases. Metastases originating from bronchogenic carcinoma chiefly create an osteolytic extensive destruction.

If the invasion of the epidural space from the primary or secondary tumors is unilateral, myelography will demonstrate a narrowing of the subarachnoid space on one side, with a possible spinal cord compression and displacement (Figures 20 and 21).[30] On lateral films, the contrast medium may have different angulations, from sharp to obtuse, depending upon the type of spinal pathologic fracture (Figures 22). If the subarachnoid space is compressed by an extensive growth of an epdiural neoplasm, the contrast medium will narrow gradually to the point of obstruction, and the spinal cord may be seen compressed and flattened, and occasionally displaced to the opposite side (Figure 23). Gas myelography delineates the extent of the epidural mass and its relationship to the bony structures of the spine and to the subarachnoid space (Figure 23). If the epidural tumor encircles the subarachnoid space, the spinal cord will remain in a normal position and its radiolucency may be more prominent on positive contrast myelograms. The margins of the filling defect can be smooth or irregular, depending upon the shape of the neoplasm (Figure 18). The opaque or the lucent column of the contrast agent may show an asymetric tapering, or the block may cause an almost horizontal, abrupt interruption to the flow of the contrast medium. Furthermore, the lower pole of the invading tumor can be seen as a multilobulated mass, or as a radiolucency with a convex, well delineated margin, However, the limits of the tumor are usually less sharply outlined in comparison with the margin of a benign intradural extramedullary neoplasm. It may be difficult, at times, to differentiate an epidural from an intradural expansive lesion on the basis of myelography alone. Clinical data, as well as the changes demonstrated on standard radiographs and tomograms, should be considered in conjunction with myelographic findings. Epidural venography can sometimes prove helpful as an additional diagnostic procedure in the evaluation of epidural expansive masses. It should be pointed out that benign lesions, such as the herniated intervertebral disk or callus, may compress the subarachnoid space, and it can be difficult to distinguish, on myelograms, this type of compression from those produced by neoplasms. Myelographic appearance of extradural masses can be summarized in the following way: displacement of the column of contrast medium from the bony structures of the spinal canal; a lateral extradural mass displacing the spinal cord to the opposite side; a concentric neoplasm compressing the cord in the central position of the subarachnoid space demonstrating a tapering deformity; a complete block caused by an extradural mass showing most frequently a transverse irregular or serrated upper margin at the level of the obstruction; root sleeves possibly having a triangular shape, or being obliterated by the tumor.[36,38,39]

The extradural location of a dermoid and epidermoid cyst is rare.[42,44,45,49] Epidermoid cysts can be of a posttraumatic or iatrogenic origin. Iatrogenic epidermoid sequestration cysts were reported in the literature following lumbar puncture or diskography. They can involve either the intradural or epidural space in the lumbar region. The evolution of these cysts is very slow and it can last for many years.[48] Cases were reported occuring 23 years following the implantation of particles of the skin at the time of lumbar puncture. Apparently, this may occur if the stylet of the needle for the lumbar puncture does not fit tightly, being narrower and loose in the needle. Epidermoid cysts of this origin can be single or multiple, differing in size from few milimeters to several centimeters in diameter. Usually, no changes of the bony structures are seen on radiographs of the spine. Myelography can demonstrate a single or multiple neoplasm, elyptic in shape, mostly located posteriorly to the disk space. The surface of the tumor is usually smooth, but it may also have a mottled or flaky appearance.[48]

IV. REDUNDANT NERVE ROOTS OF THE CAUDA EQUINA

Redundant nerve roots is a rare anatomic entity described first in the occipital and later in the lumbar region.[53-57] Gagel (1935) considered these enlarged nerve roots to be perineural fibromas (Rankenneurofibroma, Gagel).[54] Schumacher et al. recently reported a case of redundant nerve roots that he identified as a plexiform perineural fibroma of the cauda equina.[58] This lesion occurs mostly in middle-aged men and it is associated with often severe back pain, hypesthesia in the lumbar region and lower extremities, weakness, paresis, and diminished reflexes in the lower limbs. These enlarged nerve roots may cause a complete block of the subarachnoid space and induce a considerable increase in the CSF protein.[52,58] Myelograms performed with opaque contrast media demonstrate, in the lumbar region, a complete or partial block and the presence of serpentine filling defects that simulate enlarged blood vessels. These wormlike defects are not only characteristic of plexiform neurofibroma, but can be seen also in arteriovenous malformations, familial hypertrophic neuropathy (Dejerine and Sottas), and some other conditions of the cauda equina, mentioned already in the previous text. The redundant nerve roots were in some cases so similar on myelograms to an arteriovenous malformation that angiography had to be performed for differential diagnostic purposes.[58] Selective spinal cord angiography in redundant nerve roots does not yield any diagnostic information and the correct diagnosis of plexiform neurofibroma can be reached only by biopsy.[55,58] In one patient who was operated on, we had performed Pantopaque® myelography and established a partial block of the subarachnoid space at the level of L_3. Above the partial block, the contrast medium outlined large serpentine defects. At surgery, an unusual, thickened and worm-like nerve root was uncovered occupying a considerable part of the lumbar subarachnoid space (Figure 24).

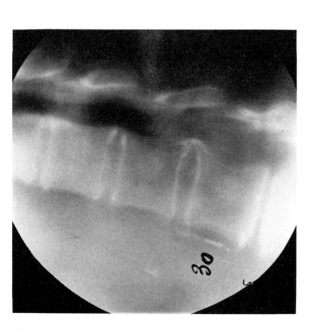

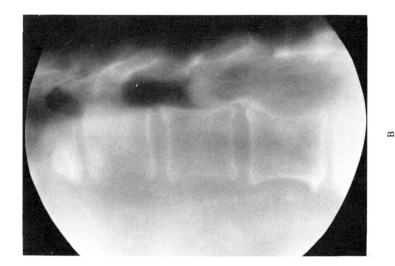

A

B

FIGURE 1(A).   A complete obstruction of the subarachnoid space at the lower margin of Th$_{12}$. The spinal cord is visualized compressed against the posterior wall of the subarachnoid space. (B) On polytomograms to the right of the midline the upper pole of the mass is sharply demarcated. The spinal canal below the block is wide. The vertebral bodies are concave and atrophic. Osteosclerotic islands are apparent in the structure of the bone. (C)   Anteroposterior projection outlines the spinal cord encircled by oxygen. A complete block is seen at Th$_{12}$ level. The spinal canal is wider below the obstruction. At surgery, a large tumor was found occupying the lumbar subarachnoid space. The tumor had the features of a giant ependymoma.

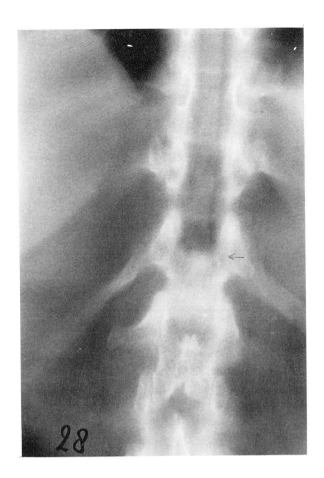

FIGURE 1C

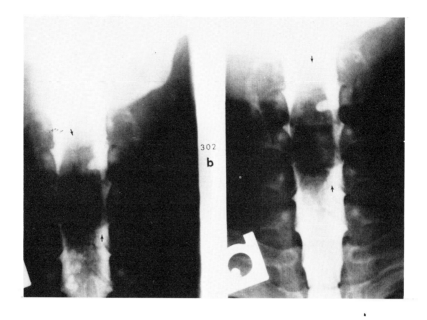

A

B

FIGURE 2(A).   Pantopaque® myelography was performed on this 27-year-old male patient with clinical signs of cervical spinal cord compression. An obstruction to the flow of the contrast was encountered at the upper margin of C_7. The contrast medium could be moved proximally through the anterior subarachnoid compartment thus outlining a large intramedullary tumor extending from C_6 to C_4. (B) In slightly oblique projections, the large defect representing an intramedullary neoplasm is surrounded by wide and prominent arachnoid sleeves encompassing the nerve roots. (C) In lateral projection, the large intramedullary mass is well circumscribed at its lower pole, and indiscernible in its proximal end. At surgery, a glioma was found (histologically confirmed) in the swollen spinal cord.

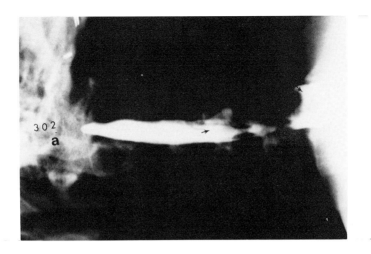

FIGURE 2C

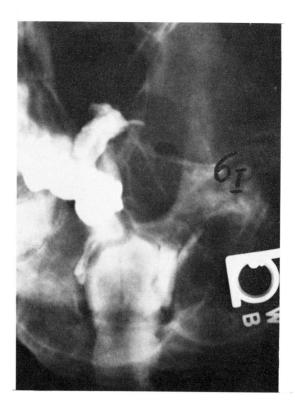

A

FIGURE 3. A male patient, 48 years old, operated upon earlier for a meningioma of the posterior fossa
came back with clinical signs of a posterior fossa space-occupying lesion. (A) Pantopaque® myelogram
shows an obstruction at the level of the base of the skull. (B) The vertebral arteries and the basilar artery
with their branches are clearly outlined. (C) Myelogram in an accentuated oblique position shows the basilar
and vertebral arteries. The contrast medium moves along the clivus but its flow is partially obstructed at
the upper margin of C_1. (D) PEG with tomography (polytome). Posterior displacement of the aqueduct.
(E) PEG reveals an enlarged pons and posterior displacement of the fourth ventricle and aqueduct. (F)
Left vertebral arteriogram in lateral view shows the area of the earlier surgery and signs of a space-occupying
lesion in the posterior fossa. (G) Left vertebral arteriogram in anteroposterior view demonstrates stretching
and displacement of the basilar artery and its branches to the right side, downward and upward. At surgery,
a large arachnoid cyst was found with a small astrocytoma penetrating through the foramen magnum into
the spinal canal up to the upper border of C_1.

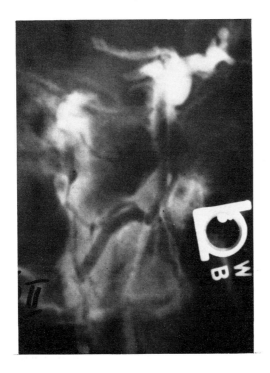

FIGURE 3B

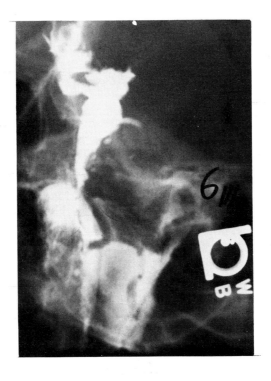

FIGURE 3C

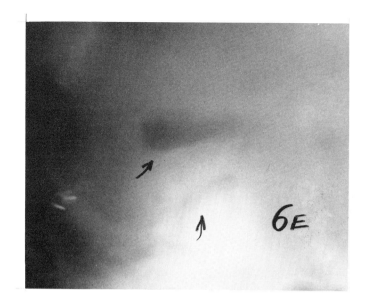

FIGURE 3D

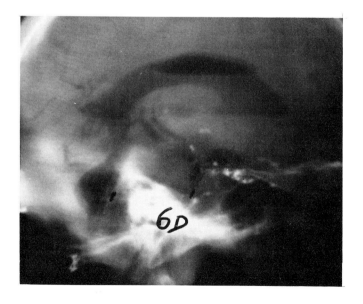

FIGURE 3E

191

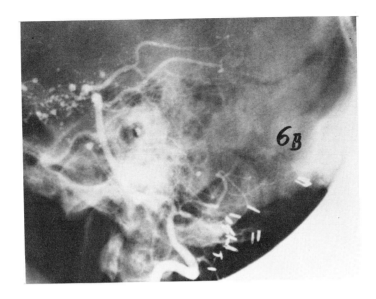

FIGURE 3F

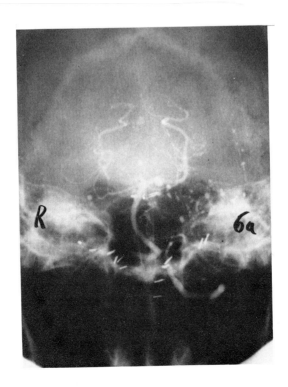

FIGURE 3G

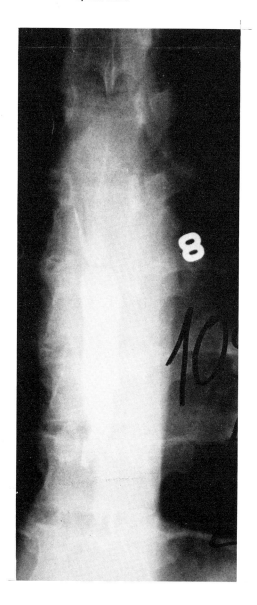

FIGURE 4.   The patient, male, 16 years old, was admitted with signs of thoracic spinal cord compression. Pantopaque® myelogram in the supine position shows a complete block at Th₈ with upward spreading of the contrast medium in the shape of the letter V. There is a radiolucent ridge dividing the upper part of the opaque column. The intramedullary lesion appeared to be of a softer consistency because Pantopaque® could partially fill the subarachnoid gutters along the widened spinal cord. The lesion was expanding the cord more in the direction of the posterior subarachnoid compartment. The radiolucent ridge was interpreted as a sign of meningeal involvement. At surgery, an intramedullary lipoma was found expanding from Th₇ to Th₄ and infiltrating dorsally the arachnoid at the point corresponding to the radiolucent ridge.

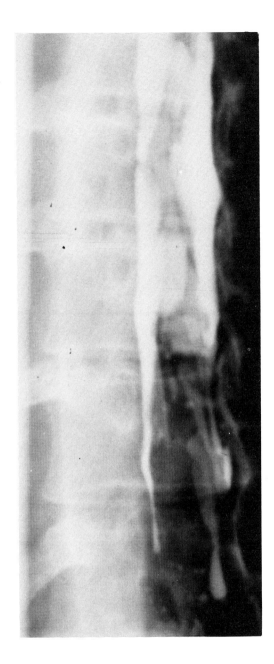

FIGURE 5. Pantopaque® myelogram represents tortuous, enlarged veins in the dorsal area in the oblique position of the patient who developed cervical hematomyelia. Acute swelling of the spinal cord obstructed the venous blood flow. The enlarged, obstructed veins can be seen in conjunction with the variety of lesions affecting the spinal cord as described in the text.

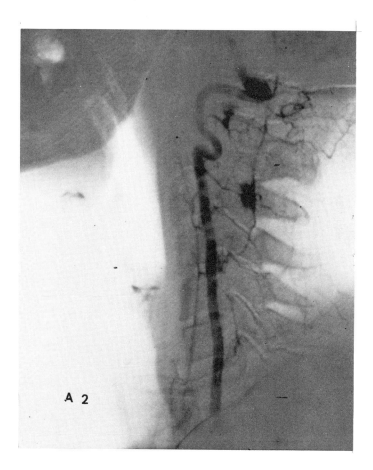

FIGURE 6.   The same patient had a cervical spinal angiography which disclosed multiple smaller and larger vascular nodules in the cervical region and displacement of arteries indicating the enlargment of the spinal cord. This type of vascular anomaly in the spinal cord is seen mainly in hemangioblastomas. Later in the text relating to spinal cord angiography, hemangioblastomas will be mentioned again. (Courtesy Dr. H. T. Moskowitz).

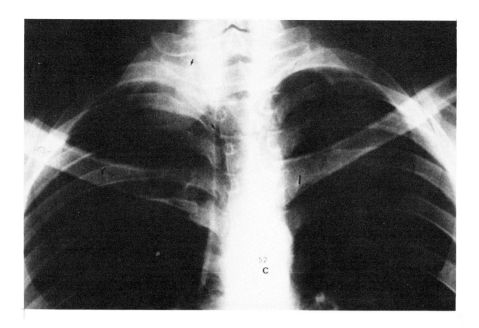

A

FIGURE 7(A). A round shadow was disclosed on routine chest examination located in the right apical region in this 28-year-old male patient (arrow). (B) Following a thorough neurological examination, a Pantopaque® myelogram was carried out in another institution. (B and C) A few weeks later, the patient was admitted with paraparesis and urinary disturbances. Gas myelography was performed and it showed a relative obstruction of the subarachnoid space at Th$_2$ level. The previously injected Pantopaque® could not bypass this obstruction. This double contrast technique illustrates the advantage of gas over Pantopaque® in such situations (arrow). (D) The double contrast myelogram indicates that the obstruction is caused by a dumbbell tumor (arrow). Radiologic diagnosis of neurofibroma was established and confirmed at surgery.

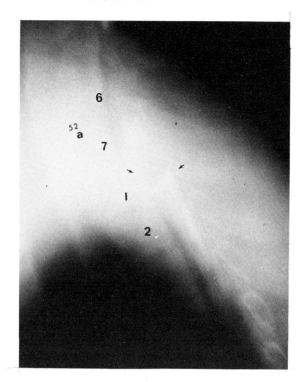

FIGURE 7B

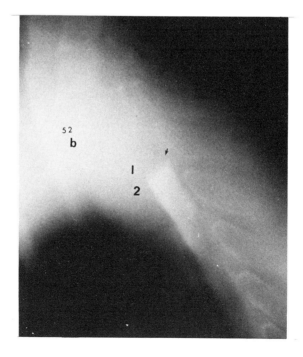

FIGURE 7C

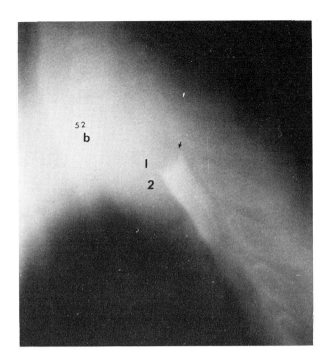

FIGURE 7D

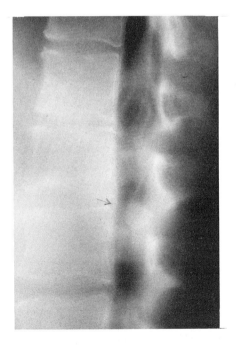

A

FIGURE 8(A).   Gas myelogram of the lumbar area shows a clearly outlined, round tumor (arrow) located in the subarachnoid space and transsected by the nerve. (B) In the proximal part of the gas myelogram, the conus with the emerging nerves of the cauda equina is visualized. The tumor was considered as a neurofibroma, later proved at surgery.

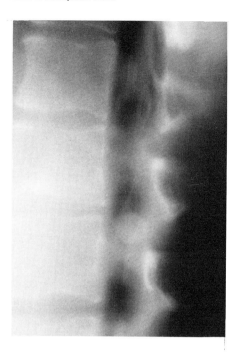

FIGURE 8B

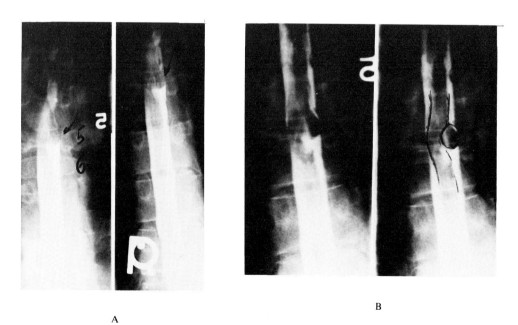

A

B

FIGURE 9.   A male patient, 23 years old, with gradually developing signs of thoracic radiculomyelopathy.
(A) Pantopaque® myelogram in the supine position reveals the sign of the cup at Th_6 to Th_5 level at the
left side with a slight displacement of the spinal cord to the right side. (B) The contrast medium encircles
the tumor from the cranial and caudal directions. The subarachnoid space is not obstructed. The tumor is
round, extramedullary, and localized posterolaterally. At surgery, a small neurofibroma was removed from
the left posterolateral subarachonid space.

199

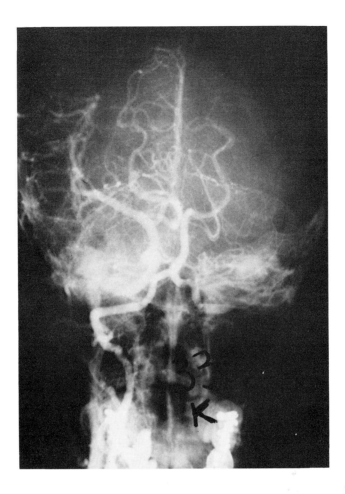

A

FIGURE 10. An 8-year-old female, admitted with clinical signs of an intracranial expansive process.
(A) Right brachial angiogram in anteroposterior shows a large neoplasm in the middle cranial fossa
expanding posteriorly. (B) The same angiogram in the later phase demonstrates a well vascularized
tumor, probably a meningioma. At surgery, a large meningioma was found and partially removed. Multiple plaques of the tumor tissue were seen extending downward into the posterior fossa attached to the
meningeal sheaths. (C) On second admittance 2 years later, the patient had signs of spinal cord involvement. The Pantopaque® myelogram discloses a small, round tumor at C_2 level on the right side. The
cervical nerve roots and the anterior spinal artery are clearly visualized. (D) In oblique views the round
defect is clearly seen. The dentate ligament and the spinal cord are clearly outlined. (E) The mentioned
defect has a multilobulated shape. The cervical nerve roots and tributary arteries are apparent. (F)
Pantopaque® was introduced from the cervical subarachnoid space into the fourth ventricle to evaluate
the posterior fossa. The fourth ventricle and the aqueduct are displaced posteriorly and the cisterna
magna flattened. (G) In the anteroposterior view, the fourth ventricle is displaced to the left by the
tumor. The patient was reoperated on and the meningioma partially removed. Diffuse plaques of the
tumor were found attached to the meninges. (H) The third admittance of the patient. Myelogram shows
a complete block at C_2 to C_3 level. The anterior and posterior subarachnoid compartments are filled
with Pantopaque®. Dorsally at the level of the block, the surface of the tumor is demarcated and the
dentate ligament is prominent. At surgery multiple smaller and larger tumors, some of them in the shape
of plaques, were disclosed. This meningioma was spreading from the middle intracranial fossa to the
cervical area in the form of plaques and smaller nodular tumors attached to the meninges.

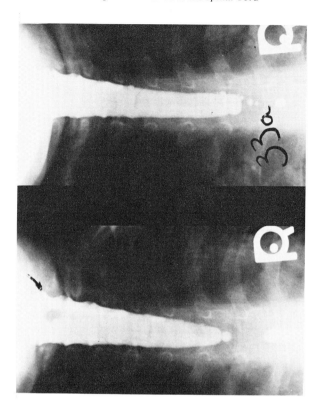

FIGURE 10C

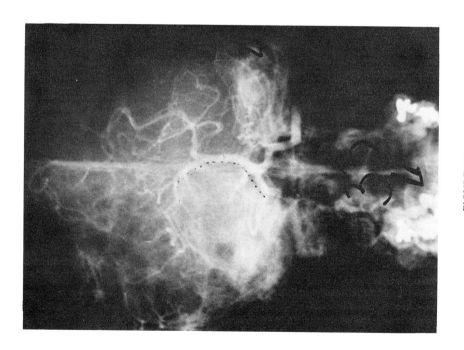

FIGURE 10B

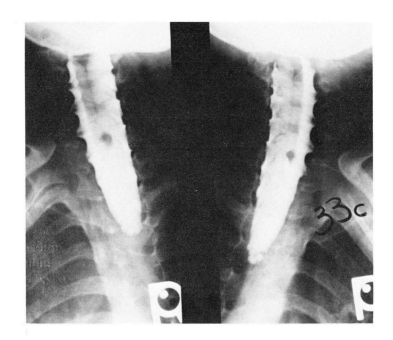

FIGURE 10D

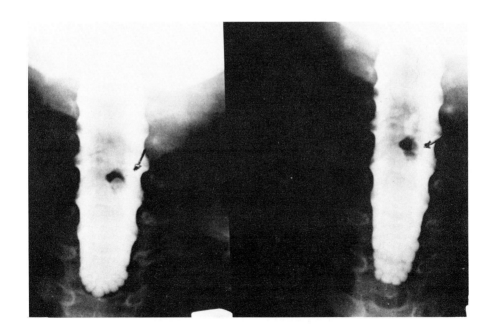

FIGURE 10E

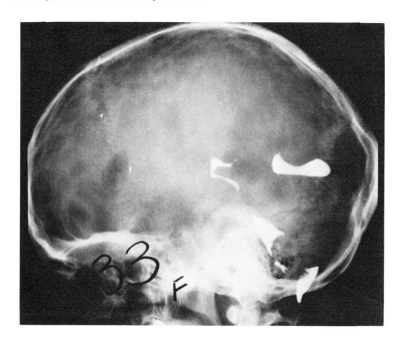

FIGURE 10F

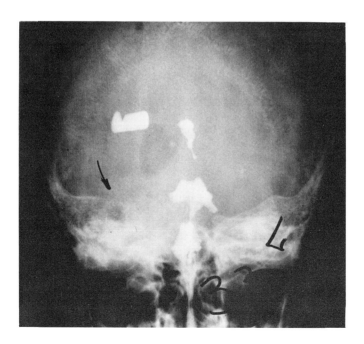

FIGURE 10G

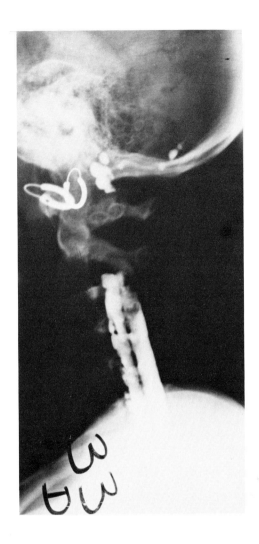

FIGURE 10H

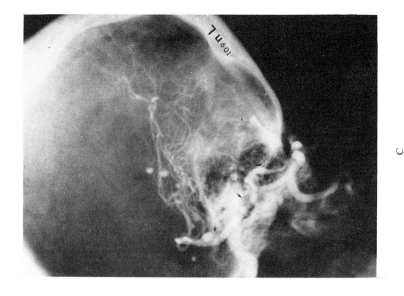

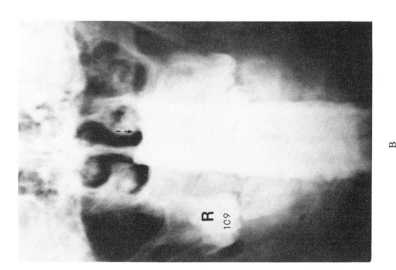

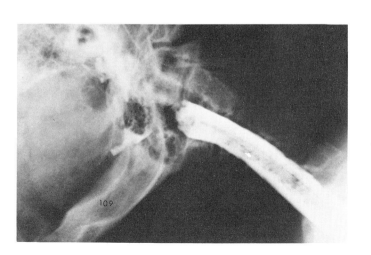

FIGURE 11. The patient, female, 39 years old, with quadriparalysis, spastic lower extremities. CSF clear, manometric study normal. (A) In the right oblique position the contrast medium stops at the level of C_1. The dentate ligament is well outlined, as well as the spinal cord and the nerve roots. The cisterna magna is partially filled with Pantopaque®. (B) In the supine position a bilobulated mass is outlined at the junction C_1 – foramen magnum. The ligamentum posticum is delineated. (C) Left vertebral arteriography: downward displacement of the inferior posterior cerebellar artery, and forward displacement of the vertebral arteries junction and the basilar artery. Surgical finding: dorsally located meningioma attached to the meninges at the upper level of C_1 protruding into foramen magnum.

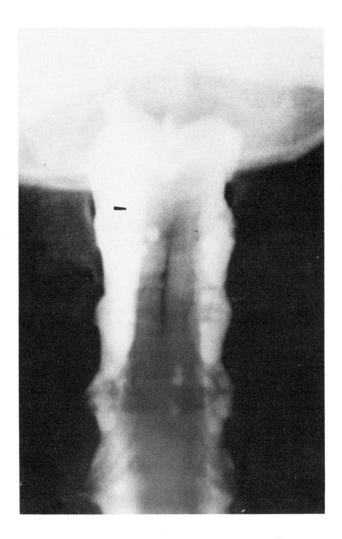

A

FIGURE 12(A).   Pantopaque® myelogram of a male, 35 years old, with signs of spinal cord compression, shows a displacement of the spinal cord to the right side at C_1 level (arrow). Widening of the left subarachnoid gutter is seen. At the level of C_4 to C_5 the nerve root and the tributary arteries are well delineated. The anterior spinal artery is seen in the upper cervical region. (B) Myelogram in the prone position shows spinal cord displacement to the right. There was no obstruction to the flow of the contrast medium. (C) Lateral supine view discloses a block at C_1 level. (D) Anteroposterior myelogram in the supine position presents a bilobulated mass at C_1 level. Globulation of Pantopaque® often occurs in the cervical region in the supine position. At surgery a multilobulated meningioma was found in the posterior subarachnoid space at C_1 level protruding through the foramen magnum into the posterior fossa. The tumor was completely removed.

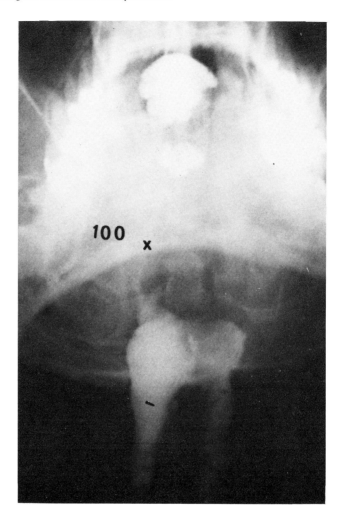

FIGURE 12B

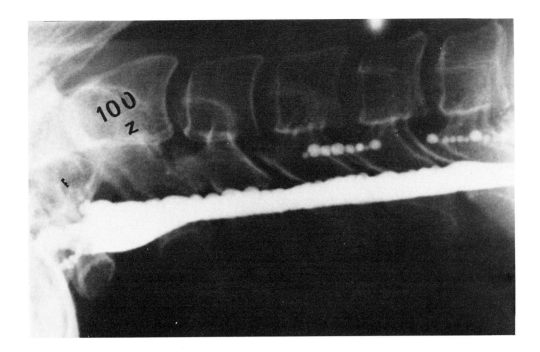

FIGURE 12C

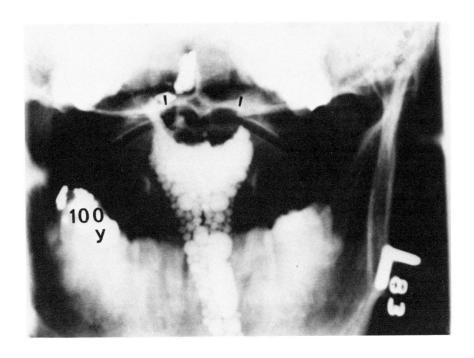

FIGURE 12D

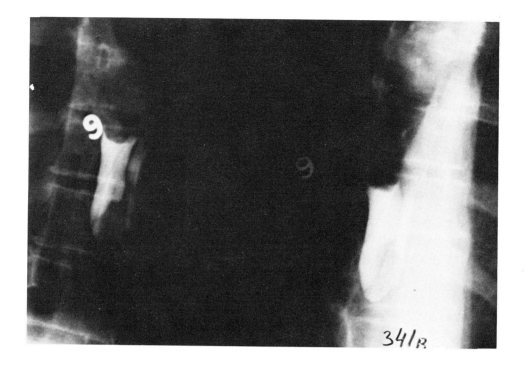

A

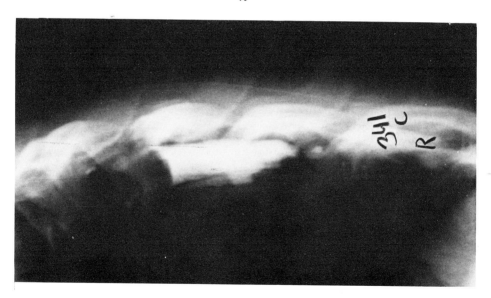

B

FIGURE 13(A).   The patient, male 37 years old, had gradual onset of radicular pain at Th_{10} level. Hypalgesia below the third vertebra. Incontinence. In the prone oblique position Pantopaque® myelogram shows a complete block at Th_9 level. The spinal cord is displaced to the right side and flattened. A stretched nerve root is seen. The sign of the cup well outlined. The level is marked with lead numbers. A small quantity of Pantopaque® was used (4 cc). Surgery: meningioma was found in the left posterolateral location, about 3 cm long. The tumor had a small attachment to the dura and came out easily. (B) Myelogram in the lateral prone position of the patient demonstrates the extramedullary location of the tumor and the ventral displacement of the spinal cord.

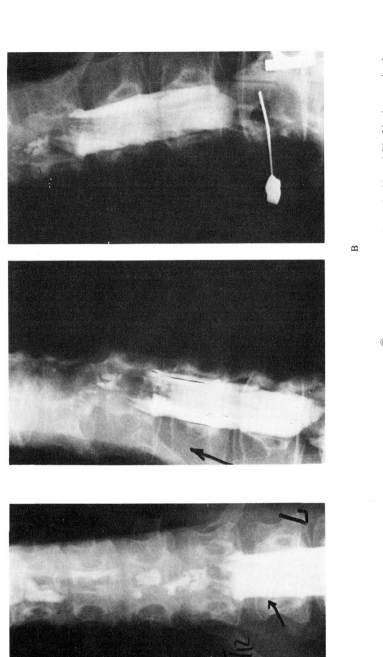

A

B

FIGURE 14. A 32-year-old woman with inconclusive clinical signs of a spinal cord disease. Pantopaque® myelography was performed. (A and B) Myelogram in the supine anterioposterior and oblique positions reveals a partial block at the Th_{12} level. The spinal cord is displaced to the right side; the left subarachnoid gutter is wider; and the sign of the cup (arrow) delineated. (C) The contrast medium having bypassed the tumor is returned caudally and it outlines the mass from above. The spinal cord is seen flattened and compressed against the opposite wall of the subarachnoid space. The reversed sign of the cup marks the upper pole of the tumor. (D) Myelogram in the lateral projection demonstrates a dorsoventral displacement and compression of the spinal cord. The sign of the cup is located dorsally. At surgery, a meningioma was removed from the posterolateral right subarachnoid space at Th_{12}.

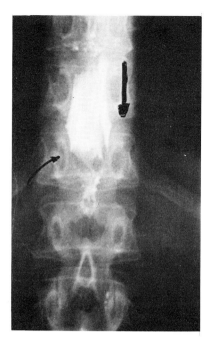
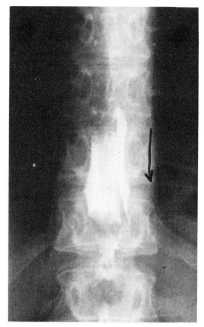

FIGURE 14C

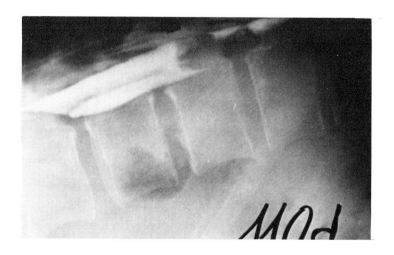

FIGURE 14D

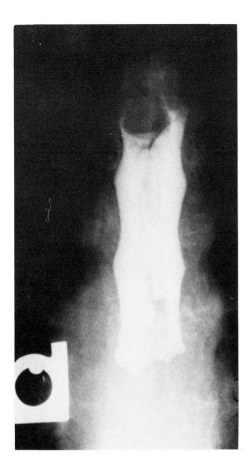
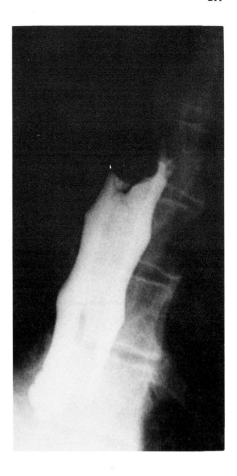

A   B

FIGURE 15. The patient, female, 60 years old, on admittance had signs of spinal cord lesion (leg weakness, spastic gait, bilateral Babinski, absent lower abdominal reflexes, absent vibratory sign, etc.). Pantopaque® myelography was performed. (A) Myelogram in the prone position shows an obstruction at Th$_5$ level with a cup sign on the left site. The spinal cord is not clearly visible because of the accumulation of the contrast medium. (B) In oblique position Pantopaque® can bypass the obstruction forming a thin streaky line. The spinal cord seems to be compressed to the right side. The sign of the cup is more evident. (C) Myelogram in the lateral view discloses a flattened spinal cord compressed against the ventral wall of the subarachnoid space. The sign of the cup is positioned dorsally to the spinal cord. The posterior subarachnoid compartment is unusually wide. (D) A smaller amount of Pantopaque® is used to outline the upper pole of the tumor. The sign of the cup is prominent. The globulation of Pantopaque® is apparent. Different metallic indicators can be used to mark the level of the lesion, the side of the patient, and the direction of the flow of the contrast medium. At surgery a 5 cm long meningioma attached to the dura was found. It was located on the left posterior side of the compressed spinal cord. The tumor was completely removed.

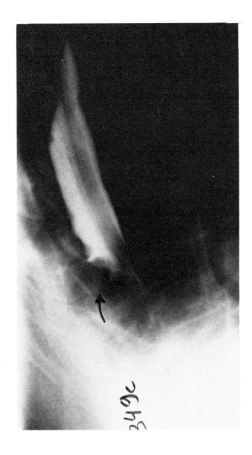

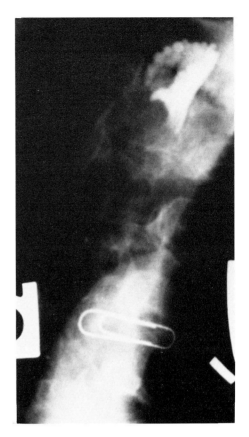

FIGURE 15C

FIGURE 15D

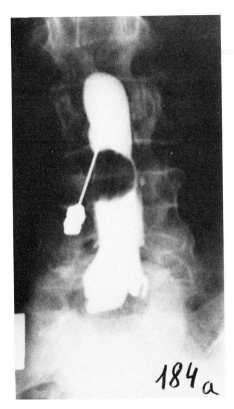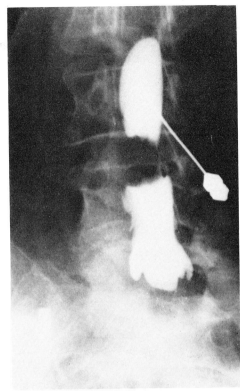

FIGURE 16. The patient, female, 74 years old, complained of a progressive low back pain of 3-month duration. Pantopaque® myelogram revealed a large, well demarcated double contour defect between L₃ and L₄. The contrast medium fills the right subarachnoid gutter and encompasses the mass. The nerve roots are displaced below the lower pole of the lesion. A herniated disk was considered in the process of differential diagnostic evaluation. However, the lesion extends below the intervertebral space, which suggests the possibility of a tumor. It was assumed that the lesion was probably a neurofibroma. At surgery, a large meningioma with abundant psammoma bodies was removed.

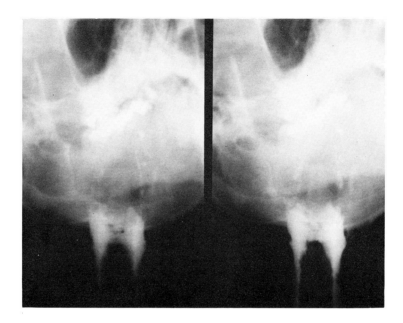

A

FIGURE 17(A). Myelogram in the prone position of a 39-year-old woman discloses a widening of the subarachnoid gutters in the upper cervical area. The contrast medium moves further up with some difficulties. (B) In the accentuated oblique position an obstruction to the flow of Pantopaque® is seen at the level of C_1. The dentate ligament is prominent. (C) Right brachial angiogram in the arterial phase demonstrates a well vascularized, sharply delineated, round tumor protruding with its lower pole into the dorsal cervical subarachnoid compartment. (D) Angiogram in a later arterial phase presents the tumor even more clearly. Small lakes of contrast medium are seen in the densely opacified neoplasm. (E) Left vertebral arteriogram clearly depicts the tumor that was, on the basis of these studies, considered as a meningioma. At surgery the tumor was found attached to the posterior rim of the foramen magnum. It was a highly vascularized neoplasm. The tumor was completely removed. The histological findings indicated that the tumor was a hemangioblastic meningioma.

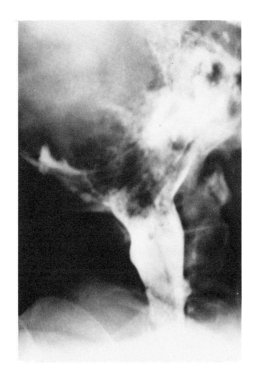

FIGURE 17B

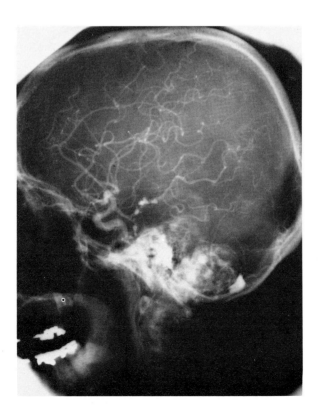

FIGURE 17C

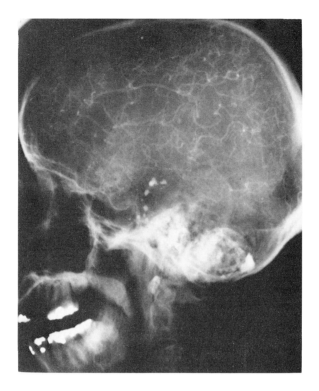

FIGURE 17D

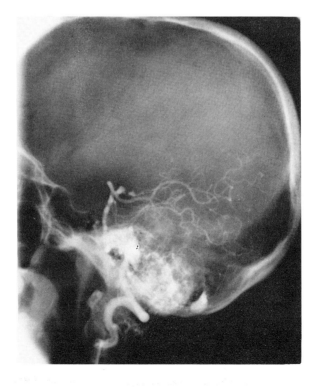

FIGURE 17E

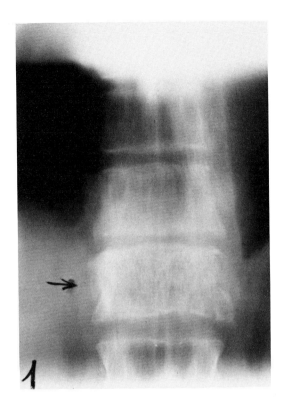

A

FIGURE 18(A). Radiograph of the Th₁₂ vertebra shows a trabecular distribution of the body indicating the presence of a hemangioma. (B) Pantopaque® myelography was performed because the patient had developed paraplegia. A complete block was encountered at Th₁₂ level; the margins of the filling defect are irregular and the spinal cord appears wider due to the compression. (C) Oblique view delineates the contour of the obstructed area. About 6 cc of Pantopaque® was used for this examination. The tumor was identified at surgery as hemangioma.

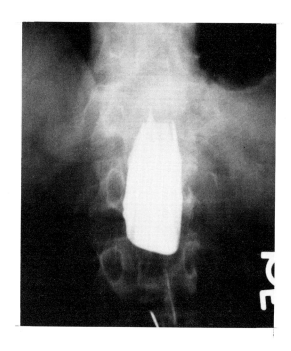

FIGURE 18B

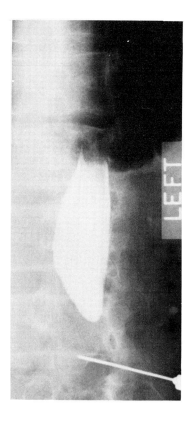

FIGURE 18C

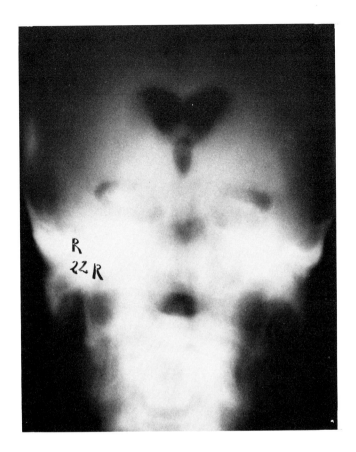

A

FIGURE 19.   Patient, female, 36 years old, developed progressive signs of a posterior fossa lesion and upper spinal cord compression. (A) Pneumoencephalography, anteroposterior view, shows clearly outlined ventricles. The fourth ventricle in the lateral projection is displaced posteriorly and the subarachnoid space dorsal to the clivus is not seen. Previously performed cerebral angiography was inconclusive. (B) Pantopaque® myelogram in the prone position shows a large defect at the base of the skull in the anteroposterior position (arrows). (C) The defect is outlined in an accentuated Trendelenburg position. (D) In the left oblique position, the myelogram shows the defect bypassed by the contrast medium. The basilar and vertebral arteries are outlined with some of their branches. (E) Myelogram, right oblique position, shows the defect and the major arteries. The large bilobulated tumor analyzed histologically was diagnosed as chordoma.

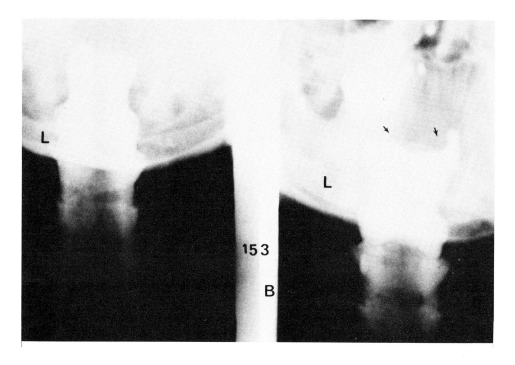

FIGURE 19B

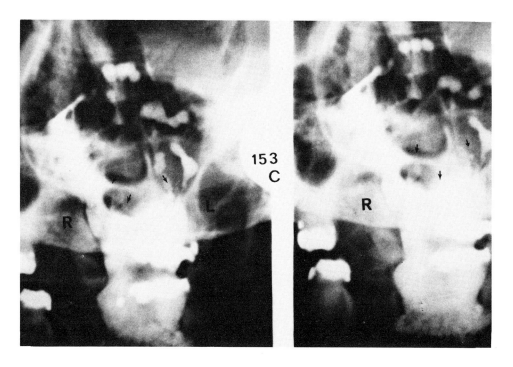

FIGURE 19C

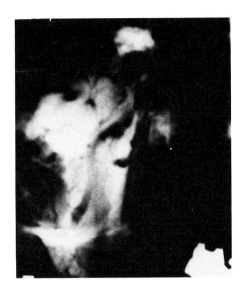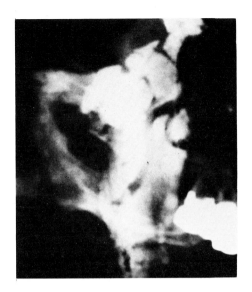

FIGURE 19D

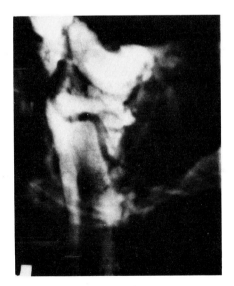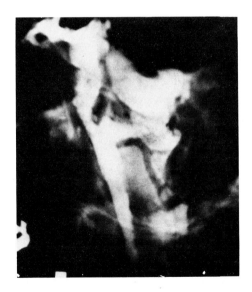

FIGURE 19E

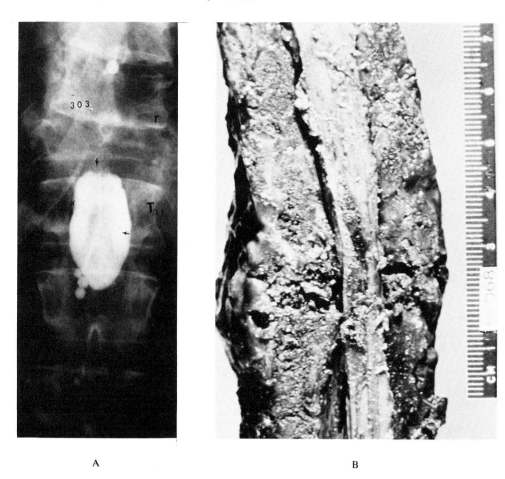

A   B

FIGURE 20.   This 63-year-old man had developed paraplegia and underwent treatment for multiple myeloma. (A) Lumbar myelogram reveals a complete block at Th₁₁ (arrows) and a collapse of the vertebral
body. The subarachnoid gutters are distended and the spinal cord compressed by the epidural mass. A small
quantity of Pantopaque® was injected (4 cc). (B) The pathologic specimen shows the extent of bone destruction and the invasion of the meninges and spinal cord by a tumor. (Courtesy of Department of Pathology,
Johns Hopkins University, School of Medicine, Baltimore, Md.).

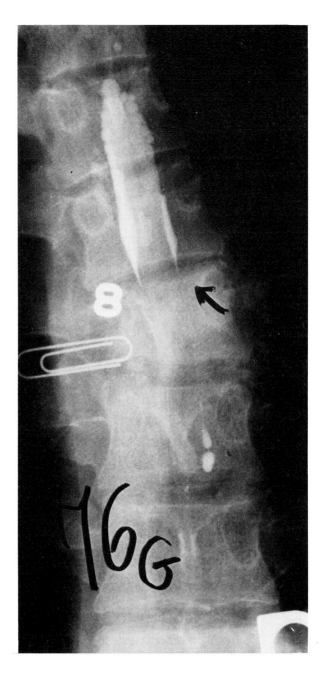

A

FIGURE 21. Patient, female, 20 years old, developed paraplegia as the first sign of lymphogranulomatosis. Two myelographies were performed. (A) First myelography was done via suboccipital instillation of Pantopaque®. The myelogram in the prone position discloses a complete block at Th₈ level. The spinal cord appears compressed and flattened by an epidural mass extending from the partially destructed Th₈ vertebral body. (B) Pantopaque® myelography following radiation therapy demonstrates a free movement of the contrast medium in the lumbar subarachnoid space. (C) The contrast medium moves freely into the cranial direction. (D) In the supine position the previously seen block is not detectable. The septum posticum is well outlined. Some irregularities are seen on the arachnoid walls at Th₈ indicating the possibility of the presence of arachnoid adhesions.

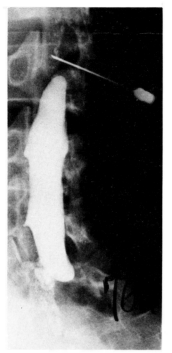
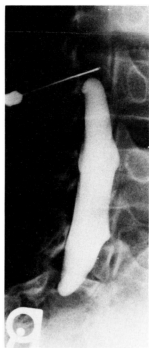

FIGURE 21B

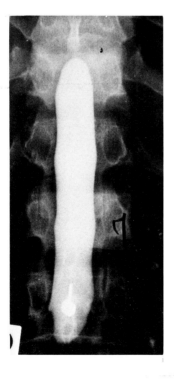
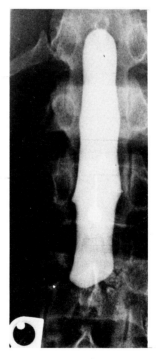

FIGURE 21C

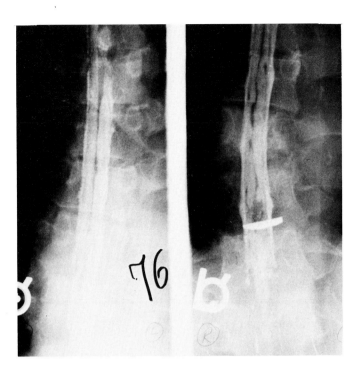

FIGURE 21D

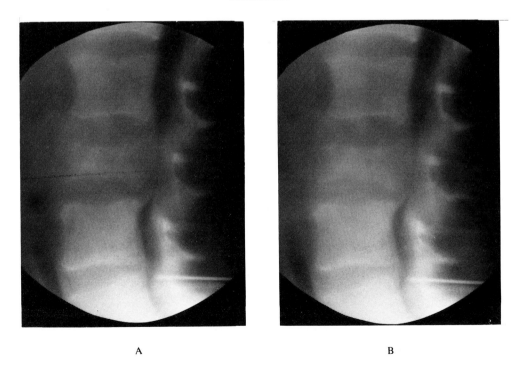

A   B

FIGURE 22.   Gas myelograms demonstrate osteolitic metastasis of breast carcinoma spreading from L_1 vertebra. The neoplasm invaded extensively the epidural space and caused a severe compression of the subarachnoid space and spinal canal. The present pathologic fracture of L_2 contributes to the reduction of the subarachnoid space. The characteristic myelographic findings of an expansive epidural process are illustrated on these gas myelograms. The distance between the objective planes of the two polytomograms was 3 mm. (Patient referred from the Clinic of Neurology, University of Geneva.)

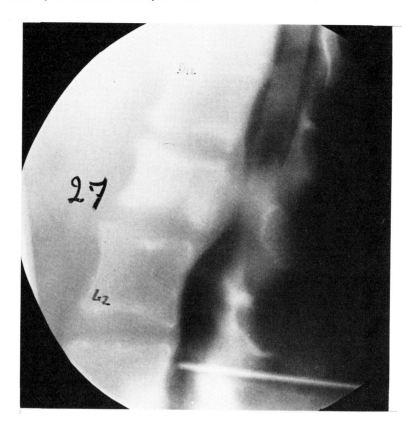

A

FIGURE 23.   An almost complete obstruction of the subarachnoid space surrounded by a mass extending from L_2 vertebra is demonstrated on this gas myelogram. The spinal cord involved in the tumor is displaced and the epidural space diffusely infiltrated. The vertebral body L_1 appears osteosclerotic. The metastasis of this breast carcinoma has the characteristics of an epidural mass, as described in the text. (Patient referred from the Clinic of Neurology, University of Geneva).

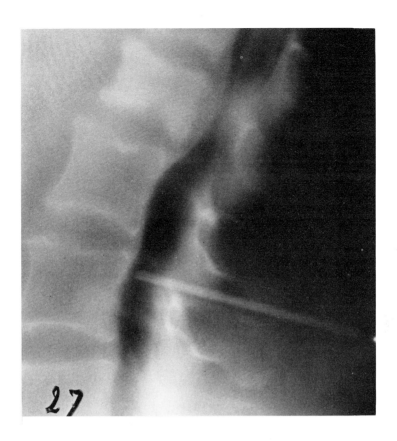

FIGURE 23B

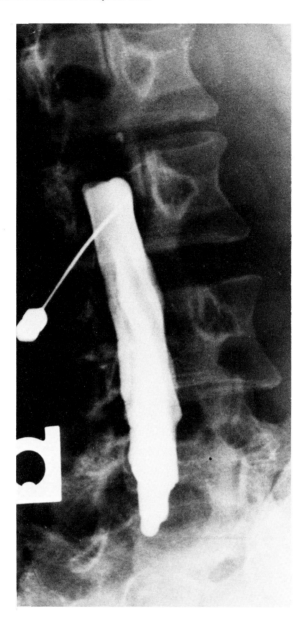

FIGURE 24.   A 27-year-old male with severe back pain had
a Pantopaque® myelography. A partial block was encountered at L₃ level with wide, unusually prominent nerves of the
cauda equina. The operative finding was redundant nerve root.

REFERENCES

1. **Phillips, T.,** An account of a tumor situated in the lumbar vertebrae of a very extraordinary size and singular appearance and which ensued from a fall, *N. London Med. J.,* 1, 144, 1792.
2. **Bailey, P., and Cushing, H.,** *A Classification of the Tumors of the Glioma Group on a Histogenetic Basis with Correlated Study of Prognosis,* Lippincott, Philadelphia, 1926.
3. **Tarlov, I. M.,** Acute spinal cord compression paralysis, *J. Neurosurg.,* 36, 10, 1972.
4. **Baker, G. S. and Mulder, R. W.,** Spinal cord tumors, in *Clinical Neurology,* 2nd ed., Baker, A. B., Ed., Hoeber-Harper, New York, 1965, chap. 33.
5. **Sloof, J. L., Kernoman, J. W., and MacCarty, C. S.,** *Primary Intramedullary Tumors of the Spinal Cord and Filum Terminale,* W. B. Saunders, Philadelphia, 1964.
6. **Russell, D. S. and Rubinstein, L. J.,** *Pathology of Tumors of the Nervous System,* 3rd ed., Edward Arnold Publishers, London, 1971.
7. **Hughes, J. T.,** *Pathology of the Spinal Cord,* 2nd ed., W. B. Saunders, Philadelphia, 1978, chap. 10.
8. **Woltman, H. W., Kernohan, J. W., Adson, A. W., and Craig, W. McK.,** Intramedullary tumors of spinal cord and gliomas of intradural portion of filum terminale, *Arch. Neurol. Pyschiatry,* 65, 378, 1951.
9. **Rasmussen, T. B., Kernohan, J. W., and Adson, A. W.,** Pathologic classification with surgical consideration of intraspinal tumors, *Ann. Surg.,* 111, 513, 1940.
10. **Till, K.,** Observations on spinal tumors in childhood, *Proc. R. Soc. Med.,* 52, 333, 1959.
11. **Tucker, A. S., Aramsri, B., and Gardner, W. J.,** Primary spinal tumors: a seven year study, *Am. J. Roentgenol.,* 87, 371, 1962.
12. **Traub, S. P.,** Mass lesions in the spinal canal, *Semin. Roentgenol.,* 7, 240, 1972.
13. **Ingraham, F. E. and Matson, D. D.,** *Neurosurgery of Infancy and Childhood,* Charles C Thomas, Springfield, Ill., 1954.
14. **Taveras, J. M. and Wood, E. H.,** *Diagnostic Neuroradiology,* 2nd ed., Vol. 2 (Part 7), Williams & Wilkins, Baltimore, 1976.
15. **Shapiro, R.,** *Myelography,* 3rd ed., Year Book Medical Publishers, Chicago, 1975, chap. 15.
16. **Furtado, D. and Marques, V.,** Spinal teratoma, *J. Neuropathol. Exp. Neurol.,* 10, 384, 1951.
17. **Rogers, H. M., Long, D. M., Chou, S. N., and French, L. A.,** Lipomas of the spinal cord and cauda equina, *J. Neurosurg.,* 34, 349, 1971.
18. **Krishnan, K. R. and Smith, W. T.,** Intramedullary haemangioblastoma of the spinal cord associated with pial varicosities simulating intradural angioma, *J. Neurol. Neurosurg. Psychiatry,* 24, 350, 1961.
19. **Brain, R. W. and Walton, J. N.,** *Brain's Diseases of the Nervous System,* 17th ed., Oxford University Press, London, 1969, 639.
20. **Perovitch, M.,** Neuroradiological approach to the diagnosis of hemangioblastomas of the spinal cord associated with hemorrhage, *11th World Congr. of Neurology,* Excerpta Medica, Amsterdam, 427, (Abstr.), 145, 1977.
21. **Sherbourne, D. H., Tribe, C. R., and Varma, S.,** Intramedullary spinal cord metastases. A clinico-pathological report of three cases, *Int. J. Paraplegia,* 2, 100, 1964.
22. **Chason, J. L., Walker, F. B., and Landers, J. W.,** Metastatic carcinoma in the central nervous system and dorsal root ganglia, *Cancer (Philadelphia),* 16, 781, 1963.
23. **Vakili, H.,** *The Spinal Cord,* International Medical Book, New York, 1967, chap. 4.
24. **Lombardi, G. and Passerini, A.,** Spinal cord tumors, *Radiology,* 76, 381, 1961.
25. **Bull, J. W. D.,** Spinal meningiomas and neurofibromas, *Acta Radiol. Diagn.,* 40, 283, 1953.
26. **Calogero, J. A. and Mossy, J.,** Extradural spinal meningiomas. Report of four cases, *J. Neurosurg.,* 37, 442, 1972.
27. **Hallpike, J. F. and Stanley, P.,** A case of extradural spinal meningiomas, *J. Neurol. Neurosurg. Psychiatry,* 31, 195, 1968.
28. **Wood, E. H., Jr. and Himadi, G. M.,** Chordomas: a roentgenologic study of sixteen cases previously unreported, *Radiology,* 54, 706, 1950.
29. **Barron, K. D., Hirano, A., Araki, S., and Terry, R. D.,** Experience with metastatic neoplasms involving the spinal cord, *Neurology,* 9, 91, 1959.
30. **Heiser, S. and Swyer, A. J.,** Myelography in spinal metastases, *Radiology,* 62, 695, 1954.
31. **Bucy, P. C. and Jerva, M. J.,** Primary epidural spinal lymphosarcoma, *J. Neurol. Surgery,* 19, 142, 1962.
32. **McKissock, W., Bloom, W. H., and Chynn, K. Y.,** Spinal cord compression caused by plasma cell tumors, *J. Neurol. Surgery,* 18, 68, 1961.
33. **Hastings-James, R.,** Melanoma of the central nervous system, *Neuroradiology,* 109, 357, 1973.
34. **Gibberd, F. B., Ngan, H., and Swann, G. F.,** Hydrocephalus, subarachnoid haemorrhage and ependymonas of the cauda equina, *Clin. Radiol.,* 23, 422, 1972.

35. **Puljic, S., Batnitzky, S., Yang, W. C., and Schechter, M. M.,** Metastases of the medulla of the spinal cord: myelographic features, *Radiology,* 117, 89, 1975.
36. **Shapiro, J. H., Och, M., and Jacobson, H. G.,** Differential diagnosis of intradural (extramedullary) and extradural spinal canal tumors, *Radiology,* 76, 718, 1961.
37. **Epstein, B. S.,** Spinal canal mass lesions, *Radiol. Clin. North Am.,* 4, 185, 1966.
38. **Sellwood, R. B.,** The radiological approach to metastatic cancer of the brain and spine, *Brit. J. Radiol.,* 45, 647, 1972.
39. **Epstein, B. S.,** *The Spine,* 4th ed., Lea & Febiger, Philadelphia, 1976, chap. 36.
40. **Reed, J. C., Kagan Hallet, K., and Feigin, D. S.,** Neural tumors of the thorax: subject review from the AFIP, *Radiology,* 126, 9, 1978.
41. **Banna, M. and Gryspeerdt, G. L.,** Intraspinal tumors in children (excluding dysraphism), *Clin. Radiol.,* 22, 17, 1971.
42. **Bodosi, M.,** Die angeborene Spinale extradurale Zysten, *Acta Neurochir.,* 23, 275, 1970.
43. **Tucker, A. S.,** Myelography of complete spinal obstruction, *Am. J. Roentgenol.,* 76, 248, 1956.
44. **Beaudoing, A., Dieterlen, M., Bost, M., Pont, J., and Pasquier, B.,** Les lipomes sous — duraux rachidiens chez l'enfant, *Arch. Fr. Pediatr.,* 29, 431, 1972.
45. **Banerjee, T., and Hunt, W. E.,** A case of spinal cord hemangioblastoma and review of literature, *Am. Surg.,* 38, 460, 1972.
46. **Dinaker, I. and Balaparameswararo, S.,** Myelographic features of spinal neurinomas, *Int. Surg.,* 57, 730, 1972.
47. **Sachs, E. and Horrax, G.,** Cervical and lumbar pilonidal sinus communicating with intraspinal dermoids, *J. Neurosurg.,* 6, 97, 1949.
48. **Pear, B. L.,** Iatrogenic intraspinal epidermoid sequestration cysts, *Radiology,* 92, 251, 1969.
49. **Hoefnagel, D., Benirschke, K., and Duarte, J.,** Teratomatous cysts within vertebral canal, *J. Neurol. Neurosurg. Psychiatry,* 25, 159, 1962.
50. **Blackwood, W. and Corsellis, J. A. N.,** *Greenfields Neuropathology,* 3rd ed., Year Book Medical Publishers, Chicago, 1976, chap. 15.
51. **Zwartverwer, F. L., Kaplan, A. M., Hart, M. C., Hertel, G. A., and Spataro, J.,** Meningeal sarcoma of the spinal cord in a newborn, *Arch. Neurol.,* 35, 844, 1978.
52. **Gooding, M. R.,** Syringomyelia in association with a neurofibroma of the filum terminale, *J. Neurol. Neurosurg. Psychiatry,* 35, 560, 1972.
53. **Cressmann, M. R., Major, M. C., and Pawl, R. P.,** Serpentine myelographic defect caused by a redundant nerve root, *J. Neurosurg.,* 28, 391, 1968.
54. **Gagel, O.,** Tumoren der peripheren Nerven, in *Handbuch der Neurologie,* Bumke, O. and Foerster, O., Eds., Springer-Verlag, 1935, 216.
55. **Gulati, D. R. and Rout, D.,** Myelographic block caused by redundant lumbar nerve root. Case report, *J. Neurosurg.,* 38, 504, 1973.
56. **Schut, L., and Groff, R. A.,** Redundant nerve roots as a cause of complete myelographic block, *J. Neurosurg.,* 28, 394, 1968.
57. **Scott, M.** Massive plexiform neurofibroma of the occipital scalp, *J. Neurosurg.,* 25, 81, 1966.
58. **Schumacher, M., Gilsbach, J., Friedrich, H., and Mennel, H. D.,** Plexiform neurofibroma (Rankenneurofibrom) of the cauda equina, *Neuroradiology,* 15, 221, 1978.

INDEX

A

M

U

V

W

X